WAVES OF PINK II

COMMON GROUND, UNCOMMON COURAGE

JULIE PERSHING

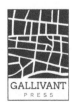

GALLIVANT
PRESS

Waves of Pink II: Common Ground, Uncommon Courage

Cover Design: Michael McCartney - DesignZ by Soup
Cover Art: Cover mermaid from original art by Corey Ford
Proof Editing: Roger Shipman
Interior Formatting and Graphics: Julie Pershing

ISBN: Paperback 978-1-947894-26-6
ISBN: Hardback: 978-1-947894-25-9
ISBN: EBook: 978-1-947894-27-3

Printed in USA

DEDICATION

This book is dedicated to the brave women within these pages who inspire us with their courage when faced with the unknown.

A breast cancer diagnosis is the fiercest battle many women will face, and they don't fight alone. Fighting breast cancer is not limited to one person, it affects families, friends, and communities.

These women are true warriors, fighting every day. They fight for their health. They fight for their families. They fight for a return to a life that doesn't focus on cancer.

They fight for you, for us.

Help us to create support and encouragement for survivors

- Share your story and picture on social media. Hold your copy of Waves of Pink using the hashtag: #wavesofpink

- Free PDF: Get a FREE full-color PDF copy of the quotes featured in the book: www.wavesofpink/bookquotes

- Leave a positive review on Amazon: bit.ly/WavesofPinkII

- Visit our website: www.pinksistas.org

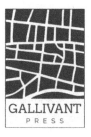

Gallivant Press is a proud supporter of Pink Sistas

CONTENTS

INTRODUCTION

One in eight women in the United States will be diagnosed with breast cancer in her lifetime. It's a frightening statistic. On average, every two minutes a woman is diagnosed with breast cancer.

They are our wives, mothers, daughters, sisters, family, lovers, and friends. Our neighbors and co-workers. They come from all walks of life, all nationalities, and all economic and social classes. We see their strength and recognize their courage, even when they don't.

The dictionary defines courage as the choice and willingness to confront agony, pain, danger or intimidation. It's the ability to do something frightening. Courage is strength in the face of pain or grief.

What kind of courage does a diagnosis of breast cancer demand? Is it the courage to face uncertainty? Is it the courage to tell your family and friends you have breast cancer? Is it the courage to face the mirror when you've lost your hair and you don't recognize your own body? Is it the courage to advocate for yourself, even when you are afraid?

Uncommon Courage. It requires discovering the courage

inside of you that grows and matures until you don't recognize it as courage—it just becomes an intrinsic part of who you are.

The chapters you will read in this book were written by women who are bonded by common ground. They share an unlikely sisterhood, and a collective desire to ensure no one fights alone. They are strong, beautiful, and wonderfully unique. Their stories highlight the challenges and triumphs of the journey. Ups and downs, joy and sorrow. The ebb and flow of navigating the life-changing diagnosis of breast cancer. Guiding us with grace—and uncommon courage.

Julie Pershing

~

Pink Sistas offers women who have been diagnosed with breast cancer no-cost retreats where they find rest and relaxation and meet others who share the same common ground.

For more information on how you can support this incredible organization, please visit https://pinksistas.org/

Make
the
days
count

CHAPTER ONE
MY NAME IS TANA
TANA HAIGLER

My name is Tana. I am a mom of three boys and a breast cancer survivor. I want to tell my story to encourage other women in their fight. Having breast cancer is hard, and even with support, you can still feel alone.

About fifteen years ago while doing my breast exam I discovered a green discharge when I squeezed my breast. I noticed it mostly on my left side, but it was coming from the right side as well. I went to my gynecologist (actually I went to her many times over the years) but she blew off my concerns, saying it was just lumpy breasts.

Fast forward to three years ago. I felt a lump the size of a small pea in my left breast, right underneath the nipple. My first thought was "well, that's kind of weird." My boyfriend Shawn worked in the medical field, and when I told him, he said, "Oh no, you really need to get that checked." I told him then I already had a feeling I knew what it was.

What I really wanted to do was ignore it, but I called my gynecologist and said, Hey, we really need to do a more thorough exam. The day of my appointment, my regular gynecologist was out of the office and I ended up seeing her PA

(Physician's Assistant). She assured me she thought it was nothing to worry about, but at the same time she advised me to have a mammogram. So, I went in for a mammogram and it was nothing: the results came back negative.

About a week later, this flash of a fever came over me. I know it was God saying, "Check your armpits." So I checked under my arm and immediately felt a peanut-sized lump in my armpit. And at that moment, I just knew—I had breast cancer.

I called my family doctor and said, "Hey, I found a lump in my armpit; I need to see you." A couple of days later I went in for an exam. He had me hold both arms out as he checked my armpit. I remember the look on his face—he was kind of scared. I told him he should not play poker; it was easy to read the worry on his face. He said I needed to have an ultrasound right away. He asked about my recent mammogram, and I told him it had come back negative.

My ultrasound and biopsy were done on a Thursday. The following Monday, I got a call at work and they told me I had Invasive Ductal Carcinoma (IDC). I knew what carcinoma was —I said WHAT? So, I have cancer? He said yes, and I'm going to set you up with a medical team who is going to take really good care of you.

I couldn't really comprehend what he was saying. I got stuck on the word carcinoma, so I just said okay. He said he would make sure the team was in place and they would start calling me to get everything set up.

I hung up the phone, ran to my coworker, and told him I have breast cancer. He hugged me. I think I was in shock—I was kind of crying but kind of not crying. I went back to my office and called Shawn and told him. I don't know what I was thinking, but I really didn't consider it to be a big deal at the time. I thought it was my cancer, and I would just deal with it. I suppose I was in denial.

The next call was to my sister Cindy, my best friend and biggest cheerleader. She said, "Oh, my gosh! You have to let me know about every appointment and what's going on." She was right there beside me from that moment on, through everything.

I knew about the cancer for about a week before I told my three boys. They are just amazing young men who have been so supportive and loving. They each dealt with my diagnosis in different ways. It was really hard for me to see the look on their faces—they were scared but didn't want to show it. Just like me, I was scared but I wouldn't allow myself to show how I really felt, and I didn't cry a lot where anyone could see. I cried in silence and in private so they wouldn't be scared. I just wanted them to be okay.

I was not in a very healthy place. I didn't know what to do with myself. Being on chemo messed with me emotionally and I was missing work. Mentally I was just not okay. I was fighting to be happy and make everybody else around me feel good because they were all scared. I hated it, but I think it was worse for everybody else around me. I had developed the mindset of "I'll get over it. I don't really want to talk about it."

I never allowed myself to ask, "Why me?" Instead, I would say thank you. Thank you that it's not my children. Thank you for not happening to my sister. My sister used to say if I could, I would take this from you. I would laugh and tell her you're not strong enough, you can't handle this.

They implanted markers when I had my biopsy. The markers were tiny pieces of titanium that would show in the scans where the cancer was in my breasts.

I was officially diagnosed with HER2 triple positive Invasive Ductal Carcinoma (IDC). Since it had traveled into my lymph nodes, it was considered metastatic. When I went on my first few doctor appointments, I shut down. I felt as if I were listening to the teacher on the Charlie Brown cartoons; I would hear a whole lot of "Wah wah woh wah wah" and not what the doctor was saying. Shawn and my sister Cindy went to my appointments with me; I counted on them to listen and keep me informed.

I did have questions. I wanted to know if I was going to lose my hair and if I could still have wine. The doctor said yes and yes. I was so pissed I was going to lose my hair! I remember I cried for about ten minutes because I worked so hard to grow my hair. But then I refocused on what was going to be the best plan for me.

After the initial visit, we hit the ground running. Within the next week I had my chemo port placed and I got a call that they wanted to start my treatment on July 4. It's not how I wanted to remember my Fourth of July, so I asked to have it moved to July 10.

The chemo port was implanted on my right side, just below my collarbone. It sat right where the seat belt goes across your body, where your bra strap lies. You could see the outline of it under my skin. I noticed people looking at the lump under my skin out of curiosity.

My first treatment was really painful. The chemo port is placed under your skin, and each time you go in, they insert a needle through your skin into the port and then the needle would lock into the back of the port. After the first three treatments, I told my doctor I needed some numbing medicine.

I learned early on to be my own advocate. I had to speak up and "fire" one of the technicians because I thought she was too rough. I don't know—maybe she was just too new. I needed someone to be gentle and take better care of me. The next tech was better, and she was there every time I went in after that. She came to know I didn't want to take a deep breath or count to ten. I didn't want to watch when she put the needle in, I just wanted to look the other way while she took care of me.

I was lucky I never threw up or got sick. I was nauseous a couple times, and everything tasted too salty. Other than the pain from accessing the port, that was probably what I hated the most about treatment.

After my third week of treatment, I started to have chemo brain. I felt like I was in a fog. I would forget anything I was told almost immediately. I would say, "Oh, my gosh, I don't even know what you said, could you please repeat yourself?" I couldn't remember people's names. It was hard to remember things for work. If I set something down, I would forget where I put it. I couldn't tell stories or remember dates. It would take me a really long time to pick a gallon of bleach because there were too many choices. My brain would go into overload. It felt almost like a short-term electrical shock.

If I had something important coming up, I was afraid I would forget. I started writing things down, or I would tell my children or my sister so they could help remind me. My sister would always call me the night before and remind me I had an appointment the next morning. When she lived near me, she would come pick me up and take me to my appointments. She lived in Bend until about halfway through my treatments and then she and her husband moved to Arizona. It broke her heart because she wasn't there when I had my surgery.

It was so scary to see the nurse put on a face shield and a full body chemical protective gown just before hooking me up to my bright orange chemo. I would watch it go down the tube until it went into my port. I felt radioactive. I used to tell my sister I felt like I was glowing.

After exactly fourteen days of treatments, I started losing my hair. I woke up one morning, and I had hair on my pillow. I cried and cried. I was a little freaked out and called my sister.

She loaned me a pair of shears that one of her girlfriends had used to shave her head. After a couple of days, I was ready, and Shawn helped me shave my head. A bottle of wine later, and it was done. I couldn't look at myself right away, it was really hard. Lots of hats and scarves helped me to cope.

Everywhere I went, I felt like a walking billboard. You can wear a beanie, but you still have that cancer look. People can still tell. My eyebrows fell out and then I lost my eyelashes. It felt like an overnight change to everything familiar about my body.

I told my doctor I didn't want to know the side effects of the medications; if I did, it would get in my head and be all I think about. We agreed I'd let him know when something happened to me or if I felt weird or different. Not knowing didn't spare me from the side effects, but it helped me not to focus on them.

The Taxol made my face feel funny. My doctor switched me to Abraxane. One side effect of the vaccine is losing your fingernails. The nails turn red and then black at the base before they lift off. I lost three fingernails.

The medication also threw me into menopause at age forty-six. I have hot flashes and can't control my body temperature. I'm hot, I'm cold. One arm might be freezing cold and the other arm is on fire. There is no rhyme or reason to it.

I went through forty rounds of chemo and twenty-five straight days of radiation. Treatment becomes your life. First you go every week then every single day to the hospital. It's a routine you get used to, and it becomes your life. And when it ends, you think, Well, now what?

They tell you you're done, and if you have any further symptoms to let them know. What does that even mean? By now you feel like you are so in touch with everything happening with your body, but then you think how do I know if it's something I should even call about?

The radiation burned my skin under my armpit and turned it black. The piece that was burned was about as big as my hand. I ended up in the Emergency Room to have it cut off because I was afraid I would snag it on something. Thankfully it has healed now, and you can't even tell the difference.

After my chemo and radiation treatments, I had a double mastectomy and the removal of seven lymph nodes (axillary node dissection).

Shawn and my oldest brother were there for me when I had surgery. Shawn's ex-wife, her mom, and daughter were also there. His ex-wife's sister had gone through brain cancer and almost died, so they understood what we were going through and were very supportive. We all prayed together before I went into surgery. I'm so thankful they were there.

I think about how unique it was to have my boyfriend's ex-wife supporting me, but I guess you just have to pick and choose your battles. This fight is not one to fight alone, and they came to stand and fight with me. They were also huge supporters at the fundraiser my best friend Angela put together for me. We are good friends to this day.

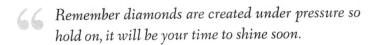

Remember diamonds are created under pressure so hold on, it will be your time to shine soon.

I love this quote about how diamonds are formed. A piece of coal goes through immense pressure to become a diamond. It encourages me and has become a metaphor for me: keep your head up and know this doesn't define you. *You are not cancer.*

I say I'm a survivor of chemo. Maybe the cancer would have eventually killed me, but it's the chemo that is toxic.

My mastectomy and reconstruction were a ten-hour surgery. My cancer surgeon completely removed my breasts, all of my breast tissue, and the affected lymph nodes under my arm. Once that part of the surgery was complete, my plastic surgeon came in to place the tissue expanders.

About a week after surgery, they begin to inject saline fluid into a port in the expanders. The expanders are small pouches used to stretch the tissue and muscle to prepare you for implants. It takes several weeks until the expanders have created enough space for the implants. The implant surgery was about four or five weeks after the expanders were placed. They remove the expanders and replace them with the implants. It was a painful process.

After my surgery I had drain tubes coming out of my side. Not only was I bald, I felt like a science project. I don't know how else to explain it. I would tell myself this is just a momentary thing, this is not forever.

At one of my post-surgery appointments, my plastic surgeon noticed a scab where the drain tube was coming out. He scolded me, as if I hadn't been showering and cleaning the wound. But I had been. Suddenly he just picked it off, and boy did it hurt! I grabbed his arm without even thinking, it hurt so bad. I think he was pretty surprised. He told me to let go of his jacket. I told him well, then don't do it again within arm's reach of me— because if I can reach you, I'm going to grab you.

I lost my job. I was struggling to pay my bills. I was prescribed Neulasta steroid shots. They are $12,000 each. There was a mix-up in the billing at the pharmacy and I found out that another medication I have to take is $323 *per pill* without insurance. When I saw that, I felt as if I were having a heart attack. I called the pharmacy and found out someone entered in the wrong number for my insurance. With insurance, it was still over $50 per pill. How do they sleep at night? It's insane. It breaks my heart and makes me angry that people can't afford their medication.

An advocate at the St. Charles Cancer Center helped me

to sign up for a program to help with non-medical living expenses, such as transportation, lodging, utility bills, and rent. The program provides you with food cards to buy groceries, gas cards to help you get to your appointments. They even helped with my electric bill.

The medical bills were staggering. I was looking at over $400,000 for my treatment. The advocate helped me sign up for a medical assistance program. I was sponsored by the hospital and they ended up paying for all my bills. I cried when I got the letter, there was just no way I could afford it. None whatsoever. It was a true blessing.

I have to go back in for another surgery because my left implant is encapsulated, it's as hard as a baseball. My choices are getting the implant removed and going flat or having fat, skin, and muscle from my back or my stomach to reconstruct. I haven't made the decision yet; I've just been living with using pads to make my breasts look even. It's a struggle to see your body go through these complications after everything else that's happened.

Sometimes I wonder if I made the right choice by getting the implants. Should I have gone flat? They found cancer on both sides, so I had no other choice than a double mastectomy. I don't know if the reason I wanted the implants was because I was vain, or because they were there my whole life and I guess I was just used to them.

After implant surgery, you no longer have nipples. Honestly it was weird to look in the mirror and not recognize my own body. After surgery, some people have their nipples tattooed, but I wasn't a candidate because my skin was too thin.

I started to research prosthetic nipples. I wanted something inexpensive, realistic looking, and made in America. I found a company called Naturally Impressive. It was started by a nurse who is a breast cancer survivor and her husband. I called and spoke with her personally to learn more. We shared our stories and I fell in love with her and her mission. I've bought three sets from her. They make me feel incredible and whole.

My advocate at the cancer center told me about the Pink Sistas Retreats. My first thought was, Oh, great, I don't want to go sit in a circle and talk to a group of women about my breast cancer or feel like I'm about to stand and speak at an AA meeting. "My name is Tana, and I have cancer . . ."

I didn't like to go to events because everyone wanted to share their opinion. You should try this naturopathic method. You should smoke some CBD. You should use these oils on your body. Have you thought about doing a cleanse? I just wanted to turn off all the unsolicited advice. So I may have had a little bit of an attitude when I showed up for the retreat. It was like, Okay, I'm here—I guess I'm supposed to do this now because I have cancer. I'll just be another one of those statistical women who goes to retreats or attends groups and bares my soul, but it wasn't like that at all.

When I went to the retreat, I was struggling with chemo brain. I would start to say something and then forget what I was talking about. At one time or another, I feel as if all of us would forget what we were saying and have to stop. But the wonderful thing about being there with people who understood was that if someone's brain was not engaging, another person would just jump in. It was such a wonderful thing.

I feel I have a good sense for what other women are feeling or going through. If they are feeling alone, I want to encourage them and take some of the fear away. Let them know that how they are feeling is not weird or strange. I probably talk too much about private things such as what your body goes through, but I throw it out there because there might be a chance it will help someone who is struggling with the silence of this horrible illness.

Honestly, the retreat was amazing. I was just so rejuvenated and full of life and on fire when I got home. I think we talked to one another just one time about our cancer journey, and the rest of the time we relaxed. We went out on the boat, and some of the ladies learned how to paddle board. At that point in my recovery, I wasn't strong enough to learn paddle boarding. I'm not a good swimmer, so I generally pass on the water stuff. But it didn't matter, we bonded. We had a weekend away from cancer.

I'm so thankful for Pink Sistas and how Deb supports women with breast cancer. I wish I had other words to express what it does for you, instead of just saying it is a group of women who have something in common. It is so much more than that. We came from different walks of life, we had different personalities. We could relate to each other, and we knew what each other was going through without really having to say too many words about it.

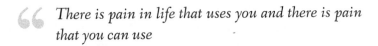

There is pain in life that uses you and there is pain that you can use

All of the things you have to deal with, and when you're finally healing, you find your new boob encapsulated. Why can't it just be easy? Why can't you go through it, get through it, and then just be done with it, to be able to say, Okay, it's all behind me. I don't know, but I guess God's not done with me. I don't know how else to explain it.

I think I went through this so I could encourage other women and help them fight. It's hard to feel alone; no one can tell you how to feel because cancer is unique for everyone, and everybody deals with it differently.

I chose to use my pain, this journey has changed me for the better, forever!

Tana Haigler

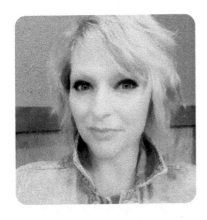

Tana Haigler lives in Bend, Oregon. She loves the outdoors, antique stores, and finding a great bargain.

She is outgoing and fun-loving and strives to build up family and friends with positive words.

Tana is a mom of three amazing boys: Lane, Cameron, and Alex. They share a once-a-month date night, usually at their favorite sushi restaurant.

After taking a year-and-a-half off to recover and heal, she is happy to be back to work as a Solutions Development Representative. Her new career allows her to fly to different destinations and meet fun, new people.

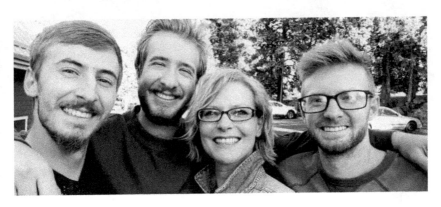

Connect with Tana
Email: aclmom@hotmail.com
Facebook: Tana Haigler Powell

Today
is
a good day
to
have
a good day

CHAPTER TWO
ONE DAY AT A TIME
AMBER CONNER

> You either get bitter or you get better. It's that simple. You either take what has been dealt to you and allow it to make you a better person, or you allow it to tear you down. The choice does not belong to fate, it belongs to you.

I HAVE HEARD different versions of the above quote throughout my life. I have tried to apply this idea to the challenges that have come along into my life. Each time I have learned something new, either about myself, about the world around me, and about other people in my life.

Without realizing it, I became a little bit stronger every time. All of the difficulties and hardships I've had to overcome led me to the moment when I got my breast cancer diagnosis. I never realized how much I learned about myself during the whole process.

I believe that if I am able to help even just one other person through their own hardship or challenge, then it was all worth the pain, suffering, ups and downs, and sickness I faced. I tell you, some of those down days were tough and I never could have won this battle with breast cancer on my own. I feel fortunate to have had so much love and support from so many wonderful people.

My husband Tony was with me through every single step of my battle with cancer. He was, has been, and still is my rock; I am thankful each and every day to have such an amazing partner. He has been in my life since the very first day we met, all those years ago in September of 1992. Our story is a miraculous love story of its very own! Every challenge along the way we faced together, and these have helped strengthen our marriage.

I remember that day in June 2018 when I got the call with my biopsy results. Deep down inside, I already knew what the results would be, but I still had a little hope my intuition was wrong. But the dreaded phone call confirmed my suspicions, the small dimpling on my left breast was cancer.

When I got off the phone, at first I felt numb and as if this moment was not really happening. But it was! I was home alone, and after a few minutes I just broke down and cried. I had no idea what was going to happen next.

When you hear the word cancer, you almost automatically think, "I am going to die." I had to remind myself that cancer is not necessarily a death sentence. My husband was diagnosed with colon cancer a few years earlier—we made it through that fight, and he is currently eight years cancer-free.

It is crazy how fast things went for me in the beginning. I have always been very diligent doing my monthly self-breast exam. I had found a little dimple during one on my exams and I saw my primary physician a month after my discovery.

My doctor and I both hoped it was just cellular changes that can happen as a woman gets older and is reaching menopausal age. She was able to get me a mammogram appointment the very same day at Providence Cancer Institute Franz Breast Care Clinic. It felt I was in a dream state as I walked from her office to the hospital where the Breast Care Clinic was located.

I was quickly escorted in for my mammogram. After the exam, I was directed to one of the changing rooms to wait for someone who would let me know if they found anything suspicious. I could tell by the technician's demeanor they had found something. I can read people pretty well without them having to say a word to me—and I was right.

Out of kindness, they squeezed me in for an ultrasound so I would not have to come back for a second appointment. I had about an hour to wait before the ultrasound; I used that time to call my husband. He helped to calm me down and reminded me of our saying, "It is not a problem until it is actually a problem. Then we will deal with it one day at a time."

The ultrasound confirmed there was something suspicious in my breast and I had a biopsy right away. The doctor that performed the biopsy did his best to keep me calm and told me it could still be something other than cancer. He assured he would call as soon as he got the results. A few days later, he called me early in the morning with the official diagnosis of breast cancer.

My official diagnosis was Stage 1 Invasive Ductal Carcinoma (IDC). It was not very big, but it was right under the nipple and the surgeon had to remove all my left breast, plus the lymph nodes. One of the lymph nodes tested positive for cancer cells, so I would have to undergo both chemo and radiation.

What? How can that be? I have no family history of breast cancer. In fact, no one in my family history has had any cancers. I went completely numb. One moment I was getting ready for work, and the next I got life-changing news. I feel so bad for the doctors who have to deliver this type of news to their patients. I had only met him one time, but I could tell he hated telling me bad news just as much as I hated receiving it.

I remember breaking down in my kitchen, crying, scared, and a little in shock as everything became real. My first call was to my husband; he had already left for work that day. Fortunately, he works close by; he left work immediately and came home because he knew I needed him. When he arrived, he scooped me up into his arms and gave me the best hug ever. He helped me calm down and reminded me we would take one thing and one day at a time. We applied this strategy when he faced his cancer battle, and we have continued to use it whenever something tough comes along.

By the end of the day, my surgeon's office called with an appointment, and I set up another with my oncologist. Next thing I knew, I was having my mastectomy, and my surgery just happened to land on our anniversary. I had a single mastectomy on my left side. I also had an expander placed during my mastectomy surgery because I planned on reconstruction.

I was afraid of how my husband Tony would react, but he is the most supportive, loving, compassionate man I have ever met. He says my scars make me even more beautiful, because they tell my story and are there to remind me how strong I really am. I feel so incredibly blessed to have his love and support. He has become a great caregiver and, believe me, that has been tested almost every day since. I am still having a lot of complications from surgeries and treatments. He has been by my side every step of the way.

I am so thankful I also have my three amazing children helping, supporting, and cheering me on throughout my battle. My mom even made the journey from Eastern Oregon to stay in Portland to offer support.

I work as an Early Childhood Educator and the families of the children I work for were so kind to me during my surgery recovery. They even prepared a meal train for my family. So many people I barely knew or were perfect strangers helped us out. I was a little uncomfortable accepting help at first. I definitely learned a great lesson in humbly accepting help from others. I realized that there are a lot of wonderful people who wanted to show their love and support in any way they could. Even with all these incredible people in my life, I still felt kind of alone at times.

My husband Tony went through his own cancer battle; he could relate a little to me and what I was going through. He treated his cancer like it wasn't even there. He kept on telling me how he got through his battle and that I should do the same.

Everyone kept telling me how brave I was. I wasn't brave; I did not choose this. Brave is when someone chooses to put themselves in harm's way in order to help others. Police officers, firefighters, those who join the military. People like that.

I thought I had to put on a smiling face all the time. I could not allow any negative feelings or thoughts to get to me. I tried my hardest to stay positive all the time, even after I started chemotherapy in August.

Chemotherapy is tough, very tough. I went through eight rounds, each round piggybacking on the last. Every round would build up in my system, making the next round harder on my body and mind to get through. I always say I would not wish chemo on my worst enemy.

During the last four rounds of chemo, I was told there was a small chance of an allergic response to the chemotherapy medications. How would I know? My body knew. Going into anaphylaxis was one of the scariest moments in my life. Almost instantly my throat started to close up and I had a hard time breathing. Afterward I was teased a little about just wanting the attention. Never had I so many medical staff run to my aid.

I finally had reconstruction surgery in February 2020. The

expander was replaced by an implant. I knew that it was risky since I did not do well with radiation. I burned so bad and there was a lot of damage and scarring. But I healed very well, and in August I finally went out and bought some nice bras and lingerie.

In September, I developed a wound on my reconstructed breast that would not heal. Between my plastic surgeon, primary physician, and express care doctor, I had four rounds of antibiotics. The wound looked better in early November, but it quickly went from bad to life-threatening. I saw my plastic surgeon December 7, and she admitted me to Providence Hospital the same day. I was prescribed three days of I.V. antibiotics, then I chose to have surgery to remove the implant. My surgeon told me I could have a new implant placed, but I did not want to go through it again.

Five days in the hospital, yet I still need another round of antibiotics. Now in the clear, I finally feel like myself again. I think my body started telling me something was wrong with the implant almost immediately. So many weird things going on with my health for months, but once the implant was removed, all the weird health issues were gone, too. My plastic surgeon was able to remove a lot of the damage inside of me that caused me so much pain for almost two years.

Once again I had to mourn the loss of my breast. Luckily, I have a wonderful husband, who loves me for me, not my outsides. He has been so supportive. He didn't want the reconstruction because he feared another surgery, but he knew I had to at least try. When I had to make the decision to try a new implant, he told me to shut my eyes, take three deep breaths, and visualize how I would feel looking in the mirror tomorrow, six months, and then years from now. That really helped. I realized that I am and will be happy without a breast—and I am!

I didn't comprehend how much the infection affected me,

physically and mentally. The prescribed drugs had some bad side effects, but now I am off all the medications, and I feel like myself again. "I am glad to finally have my wife back," says Tony.

Now let me tell you about how Pink Sistas came into my life. Just like everything else, my introduction to Pink Sistas, Deb Hart, and everything they do came quickly and out of the blue. With my permission, my mother gave my number to a recently diagnosed co-worker. I received a phone call from Bradley, now a member of the board who does a lot of volunteer work for Pink Sistas. Briefly, she told me about Pink Sistas, and the amazing retreat Deb had just hosted. I could tell by her voice and description that her experience was life-changing. Immediately after, I was on the phone with Deb Hart. You can hear and feel her radiant energy! She informed me about the who, what, when, where, and hows of Pink Sistas. She had one opening for the retreat the following weekend, and I signed up to go right then.

A few hours later, I expressed some doubts to my husband about attending the retreat. I had just completed my second round of chemo and lost all my hair. My third round would be just a few short days before going to the houseboat on the Columbia. I wouldn't know anyone. I would be feeling ill due to my recent treatment. My husband convinced me to go, so I did, though I would be out of my comfort zone.

The day of the retreat, my husband dropped me off at the houseboat marina. He gave me a huge hug and a kiss and said to have fun, relax, and to enjoy the little break I was getting from my usual routine. I grabbed my bag and headed down the walk-way, following the signs leading to Deb's houseboat at the very end of the dock.

I walked in and followed the voices up the stair to the main living area and kitchen. Right away I received a warm welcome from Deb and the other guests. My nervousness was short-lived. That weekend was so wonderful.

First, I got to meet some amazing women, each with their own personal experience with breast cancer and in various stages of their battle. Some, like me, were in treatment; others were out. It was great to hear everyone's story and experience. I was able to use so much of what I learned from them in my own battle.

Second, Deb was an amazing host and took great care of me and all the guests. The food was delicious. The weekend was filled with fun activities. Painting wine glasses and making jewelry. A fun boat ride along the Columbia River. Paddle boarding and kayaking. Yoga outside on the dock was amazing! I learned so much more about what Pink Sistas is all about, firsthand.

When the weekend was over, I felt refreshed and relaxed, which gave me more strength to endure the rest of my treatments and to win this round. I connected with some amazing women and made new friends.

I continue to be involved with Pink Sistas. The organization is run entirely by dedicated volunteers who do this out of the goodness of their hearts, especially Deb Hart!

There are several events planned throughout the year. The biggest is their annual fundraising auction (both live and silent), an amazing event with food and live music.

The money from the auction and other fundraisers provides retreats to women diagnosed with breast cancer, at absolutely no cost to them. Pretty amazing, to be able to attend one of the retreats without having to worry about cost!

Pink Sistas means so much to me and to so many others. I've received so much from them: sisterhood, advice, encouragement, strength, and most important of all, love!

Amber Conner

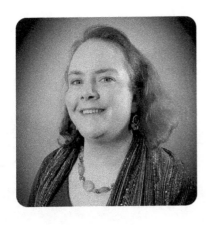

Amber Christine Conner was born and raised in the Pacific Northwest, where she developed a love of nature and the outdoors.

Oregon, Washington, and the surrounding areas have a wonderfully diverse environment that provided many opportunities for camping, hiking, rafting, sledding, and so much more.

Amber met her husband, Tony, when she was sixteen years old. They have been inseparable since the day they met, for almost thirty years now. If there is a thing as love at first sight, it happened to them. They are definitely soulmates!

Amber and Tony raised three children, their son Taylor, and daughters Kayla and Alexis. They have each grown into incredible adults. They also have two grandsons and a granddaughter. Her children and grandchildren are her world. She loves her family unconditionally and gives her whole heart to them.

She felt blessed to be a stay-at-home mom after the birth of her youngest child. Amber earned her degree in Early Childhood Education during the time she was home with her children.

Her passion is watching and helping young minds develop and grow. She feels fortunate to have a brief part in the early years that help them to mature into adults.

Connect with Amber
Email: mrsamberconner@gmail.com

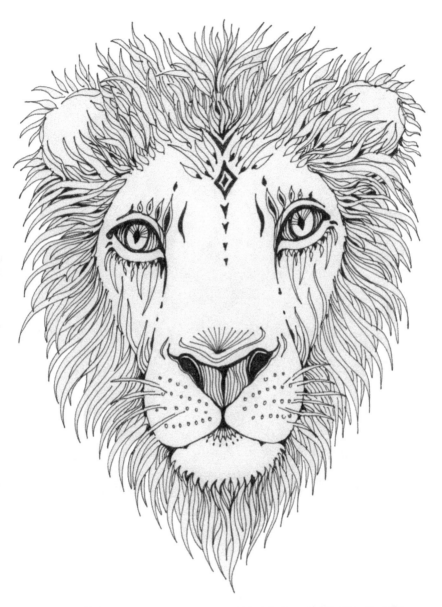

COURAGE IS BEING AFRAID,
BUT GOING ON ANYWAY

CHAPTER THREE
STRONGER FOR THE JOURNEY

MIRANDA BRENNAN

Perfect! For my weekend off I had decided to travel to Southern Oregon to see my parents. Working retail, you rarely get a weekend off. With three kids ages seventeen, eleven, and eight, I definitely didn't get time alone or to take a trip by myself. I was looking forward to some quiet time and shopping with my mom.

I made sure to pack enough pajamas. I had been sweating myself out of bed, often changing two to three times a night. My doctor had assured me it was normal to have night sweats. At thirty-nine, she said, I could be going through peri-menopause. Oh, goody!

Once at Mom and Dad's in Myrtle Creek, we did our normal visiting, then out to lunch—and of course a trip to Macy's! For once I was excited to shop as I had dropped from a size ten to a size four; and for the first time, I felt pretty good about my body. I took numerous items into the dressing room to try on. Including bras—even "the girls" had shrunk.

While changing I glanced in the mirror. I had not noticed before, but my right nipple was an odd shape. Weird. Maybe it was just squished from being in a bra all day, though my other nipple seemed normal. I put it in the back of my mind, though I had thought I had felt a lump for many months now. Almost a year! I ignored the lump, as I had just had a physical and my doctor didn't feel anything out of the norm.

The next day in the shower I did a self-exam. I normally did them around my period, but since I had it on my mind, I figured I might as well. Sure enough, there was the lump I had been feeling. Bigger this time. Pea-like and very hard. After my shower I looked in the mirror and found that not only was my right nipple a weird shape, it was also pulled downward and had a pucker at the bottom part of my breast. I asked my mom if she would look at it and tell me what she thought. Her reaction was that I get it checked out as soon as I got home. It did not look normal. It was a long three-hour drive home that Sunday at the end of July.

Monday morning, I called and found out my doctor would be unavailable for a few days, but I could get in that day to see the nurse practitioner. Mind you, I had not told my husband anything at this point, as there was nothing to worry about.

The nurse did the exam and sure enough, she felt the lump right where I told her it was. She also saw the puckering of the skin. I also told her of my horrible night sweats, which she found interesting.

She made a call for me to go right away to have a mammogram. This was my first, as I was told I was too young to have one, even though cancer ran in my family. A melanoma had metastasized to my birth mother's brain. That didn't merit having a mammogram at the age of thirty-nine. They didn't do routine mammograms till you were in your fifties or sixties.

At this point, I called my husband and he met me at the clinic. After my mammogram they sent me for an ultrasound. As the tech ran the wand over the lump, I could see a bright white spot that looked like a spider. She took measurements and pictures, then stepped out to see if the radiologist wanted to take a look. My husband and I held hands while we waited for what seemed an eternity.

Once the radiologist introduced himself, he reviewed the pictures. He ran the wand over my breast again. He tilted his head and kind of frowned. I asked what he saw, he sighed. He told us, "Well, I cannot tell you it is cancer. But I can tell you it doesn't look good. I'm sending you to a surgeon for a biopsy." I bit my lip and refused to cry.

A few days passed before I could get into the surgeon. In the meantime, I met with a cancer coordinator and found Oregon had a program for breast and cervical cancer patients who, like myself, were uninsured. Dollar signs ran through my brain. Every scan, doctor, or specialist had a co-pay, draining the bank account. I started to put a price on my health.

I had called my parents and told them the scheduled date of my biopsy. They wanted to be with me. Party in the biopsy room! It was a full house with Mom, Dad, and my husband all there, but I appreciated the support. The doctor said it would be a few days for results.

I went about my normal routine, walking in the morning to clear my mind and lift my spirits. It was a beautiful day in August by this time and I could feel the Indian summer of Central Oregon coming on. Halfway through my walk I got the call from my doctor. "It is cancer," she said. "Are you okay? Do you have anyone with you?"

"No," I said, "I'm walking." Not much I could do about it right then, so I planned to just finish my walk. She said she would set me up with my surgeon and an oncologist.

The size and type of tumor would determine my course of treatment. My surgeon felt the tumor was small enough we could do a lumpectomy and save the breast.

My parents parked their motor home in my front yard to be

here for me. The surgery was done in late August. The tumor and seventeen lymph nodes were removed, seven of which were positive with cancer. During the first surgery they did not get clear margins, so I had another surgery to make sure it was clear of cancer.

My tumor finally had a name. Stage III, HER2 positive, PR negative, 2.5 centimeters. In layman's terms, my tumor was fed by estrogen.

Next came oncology. My oncologist and I did not hit it off well at first. He was a matter-of-fact guy and didn't coddle or sugarcoat anything. I felt cold, unseen, and unheard. He prescribed six rounds of chemotherapy (Taxotere and Cytoxan) every three weeks, followed by six weeks of radiation.

My oncologist told me that fourteen days after the first treatment I would start to lose my hair. Boy, that was no lie! He had it pegged—to the day—and it fell out in clumps. At this point, I had my husband shave it. We started with a Mohawk, which my boys thought I should keep. Shaving off the Mohawk he left a tail, like people grew in the eighties! He offered to color and braid it. Yuk! So, there it was, I was bald, but my boys and husband also had shaved heads, so I was definitely not alone. I had two wigs and some super cute hats.

Every round of chemo left me a little weaker, more lethargic. I never threw up, as I would have the Neulasta shot after chemo, but nothing tasted good and I was always queasy. I lost fifteen pounds during chemo and looked quite ill. It's interesting that you seem fine until you lose your hair, then it really hits home.

I learned to love my oncologist for his matter-of-fact ways. I knew what was to be done, and how my body might react. I cried every time he walked in the room, and for being a gruff old guy, he got me.

I didn't know any other women going through treatment at

the same time I was. In the chemo lounge were other people getting their treatments, but I pretty much kept to myself. One time, there was a couple who came in to play music for us. I teased that my friends should come down to the chemo lounge where there is live music, and they serve a fabulous chemo cocktail!

I felt disconnected during radiation and went into a deep depression. My mother-in-law went with me every day, and her love and support kept me going. I saw a psychologist who helped me with medication. But I still felt alone on this journey. There was no one my age during chemo or radiation.

Time passed, my hair grew back kinky curly, and I finally knew what color my hair actually was, considering I had colored it for years. It was summer again, and I was back to walking and taking my boys to baseball. Normally, I would take on the role of "team mom" and organized snacks for the games. That year I was too self-conscious. I didn't feel outgoing and wanted to just disappear. I hated my short hair, lack of energy, and self-pity. I didn't want anyone to know I had cancer.

They say people will come into your life when you need them and that is just what happened. One day, during baseball practice, I saw a gal, younger than me, with a pretty pink ribbon chair. I eavesdropped on her conversation with another gal, who was about my age. Come to find out, they were both breast cancer survivors. I had found my people!

Needless to say, we became good friends. We swapped stories of treatment, losing hair, losing breasts, implants vs. lumpectomy. I was alive and God had sent me these two wonderful women. I was no longer alone on my journey, nor were they. And to think it happened on a ball field, where our boys all played together.

One of the ladies worked at the hospital and had connections to resources and events for cancer patients and survivors.

There was a three-day no-cost retreat coming up in November, put on by Pink Sistas, with hostess Deb Hart, for women diagnosed with breast cancer. We would be catered to and able to relax and connect with other women in different stages of their breast cancer journey.

We drove to Ty Valley, near Maupin, Oregon, a place I had never been to. We drove by a lake to a sign that said Pink Sistas. The house was a beautiful two-story colonial with a wraparound porch and welcoming rocking chairs. So inviting, it was like a storybook.

We arrived just about dinner time, so we did introductions and sat down to a wonderful home-cooked meal. While we ate, we each told snippets of who we were, how we were diagnosed, and a bit of our journey. After dinner Deb cleared and cleaned up after us. I offered to help but she said it was my weekend to relax, unwind, and feel whole again.

We explored the beautiful house, and every bedroom had a theme. Each had a couple of beds so guests who came together could stay in the same room. Once downstairs, we all settled in and Deb told her story. One of loss and heartache and beating breast cancer and beyond. She was not only surviving but thriving with a goal and purpose in life with Pink Sistas. I wholeheartedly admired her for that. I had been having my pity party for way too long. So again, I had found more of my people.

I told them how I had been doing chemo care packages for our cancer center in Bend, Oregon, during Breast Cancer Awareness Month in October. Come to find out, one of the guests at the retreat had received one of the packages. It was a little gesture to give those going through chemo hope and support.

On Saturday morning, we took a walk, looking over the lake and the lakefront houses. What a beautiful calming place to have a retreat. I opened up about my experience with breast cancer more than I had with anyone. It felt safe, because these ladies got it and understood what I was talking about and feeling. I came away from the retreat refreshed, rejuvenated, and ready to thrive not just survive this disease. I felt I had more meaning than that!

In the afternoon we did some jewelry making, which gave us another chance to chat about our journeys. I was given a lap quilt, made by a volunteer for Pink Sistas, and wouldn't you know it, I was so relaxed I fell asleep and took a little nap.

Though I did not stay in touch with everyone in the group, I did find a true friend in Deb Hart. Her Pink Sistas mission made me want to be a better survivor. To help and encourage other women who feel alone when they are going through this tough time and learning to live again. I took home more confidence than I have had in a long time.

I was living life on life's terms and things were good. My girlfriend group grew, and we all had that one word in common. Cancer. Whether it was breast, brain, skin, we all had the "big C" in common. We gathered for birthdays, holidays or just to hang out. We also attend an event every year where we dress in costume and do a 5k. It's something we look forward to doing each year, and we won "most spirited" on more than one occasion.

Years passed, my kids graduated, and my daughter got married on Maui, on our wedding anniversary. We spent our 28th anniversary and our daughter's wedding day together on Maui. It was beautiful, and cancer was the farthest thing from my mind for the first time in eight years. We were there to celebrate my daughter's marriage, and we did just that!

In 2019, I was forty-nine and planning to do my "Big 50" birthday somewhere fun. But as luck would have it, life had different plans.

I herniated a disk in March and had to have surgery. In May, I had a mole removed that had turned into a melanoma. There it is again, the C-word. Over the years, I have had precancerous moles removed here and there. Not only is melanoma in my genetics, but I was a teen of the '80s where tanning beds were the best twenty minutes a girl could have on a cold day. But in all honesty, it did not scare me like breast cancer did.

In July, I started a new job in the front office of a physical therapy center. It was an awesome job, and I was excited to get out of retail. Also very conveniently located to the radiology clinic, I could have my scans done and return to work.

I had my mammogram in January and an MRI in July, just to keep an eye on things. It's been ten years, so I was not too worried about breast cancer. It crossed my mind, yes, the thought will always be there. However, I did not live in fear of it.

But this MRI was not clear. The MRI picked up a spot in my right breast again. This time to the inner left side of my breast, against the chest wall. A biopsy was scheduled for the next week. Just as I was adjusting and getting to know my new job, I was hit with cancer again.

I should have been glowing after all of the radiation from the MRI, CT scan, mammogram, and a second CT scan, each procedure an attempt at trying to get a biopsy of this tiny cancer that had grown enough to be seen only six months after my previous scan. Finally, they were able to get the biopsy, and this time it was Triple Negative, a more aggressively growing form of cancer than I had before. This left me with pretty much one option, mastectomy. I chose bilateral mastectomy because I did not want to find myself in this position ever again.

My surgeon had a hunting trip to Alaska planned in two weeks, so I was scheduled for surgery on September 11. Funny thing, the first time I had surgery the same thing happened. He had to rush my appointment because he was going hunting. It was quite the coincidence; my cancers were almost exactly ten years apart. If I did not love his bedside manner and trust him as a breast cancer surgeon, I would not have trusted the process.

Next up was meeting with a plastic surgeon to find out if I could have breast implants done at the same time as the mastectomy.

Unfortunately, because I had already received radiation on the right side, the plastic surgeon said I was not a candidate for breast implants without the risk of infection. So I decided to wait to do a DEIP flap procedure, where they take fat from your belly and put it into your breasts. Hey, a tummy tuck *and* new tatas! It has been a year now since my mastectomy, and I'm still waiting to do it. I do not like being flat-chested or wearing prosthetics. It feels fake and uncomfortable, though eighteen hours of surgery is not something I'm in a hurry to do.

In the meantime, after my surgery in September, I celebrated turning fifty on October 14 with one of my survivor-sister best friends. We had a great time on the Oregon Coast, where you can wash your troubles away in the sand. I may not have had the endurance to walk the beach as much as I wanted. But this trip we took several shorter walks in honor of my birthday. My friend and I will continue our tradition, going to the beach in October each year, hunting for glass floats, getting the giggles, and relaxing to the sound of the surf.

Even though I have been sliced, diced, poisoned, and fried, I am still here. Life is a little sweeter, the sky is bluer, and my love for my family, friends, and Survivor Sisters, has never been stronger. I help others when I see a need and I am able to do my part to make a difference.

I am a warrior in pink, a survivor! Stronger for the journey and thankful to be given this life to live, grow, and appreciate.

Miranda Brennan

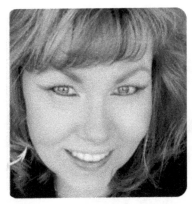

Miranda Brennan lives in Central Oregon where she and her husband of thirty years, Jeff, have raised their three children.

Her story began when she was just ten years old and lost her mother to cancer.

Miranda grew up in the foster care system. She has not only overcome a difficult childhood, but she has grown into a strong woman and thrives despite her early circumstances.

She is a member of the "one-in-eight" statistic of women who receive a diagnosis of breast cancer in their lifetime. Miranda's diagnosis came at age thirty-nine, with a recurrence at age forty-nine.

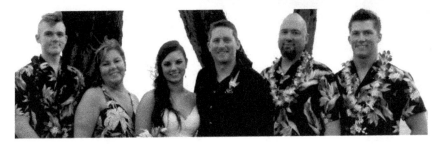

Connect with Miranda
Email: omandi3@gmail.com
Facebook: Miranda Brennan
Instagram: @omandi69

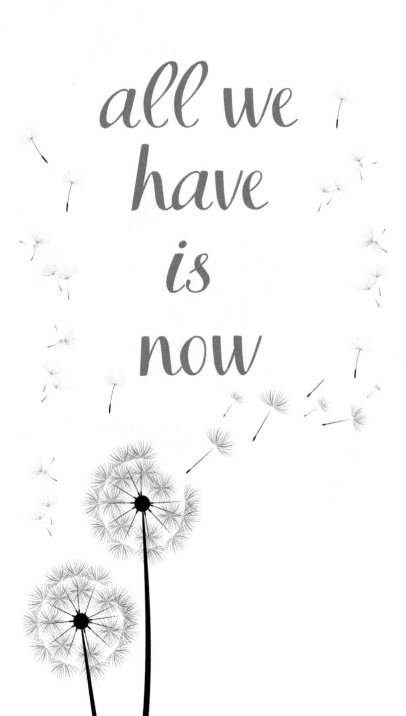

CHAPTER FOUR
A YEAR TO REMEMBER
LAUREN OMAN

HERE WE ARE. It's 2020, this is going to be the best year, a year to remember. Well, I got one of those statements correct.

JANUARY 23, 2020

Happy 40th birthday to me! Wow, forty . . . what should I do to celebrate this milestone? I know, I'll get my first ever mammogram. It's what you're supposed to do when you turn forty, right? In hindsight, I am so happy I decided to get one. I didn't know at the time, but my whole year was about to change.

FEBRUARY 28, 2020

It's mammogram time. I had heard stories about mammograms being uncomfortable or even painful so I was a little hesitant, but the nursing staff was very polite and reassured me everything would be okay. They were very nice and described the whole process as it went along. It ended up being a piece of cake. No pain, no discomfort.

Once the mammogram was finished, I asked the technician if she saw anything on the scan, even though I knew she couldn't tell me anything. She said sometimes with dense breasts, which I had, extra imaging was sometimes needed. I didn't think much of it, just a mental note to be prepared—I might have to come back for some more images.

Three days later, I received a call and indeed, they asked me to come back for another mammogram because the radiologist had noticed some suspicious areas on my left breast. Most likely calcifications, but they wanted to make sure to rule everything out since I had thyroid cancer two years ago.

MARCH 6, 2020

My second mammogram visit for the targeted areas of suspicion went just like the first appointment, very smoothly. As they suspected, it was calcifications. A lot of women have them, so again I didn't worry. Three days later, my results were in. The areas looked suspicious enough to warrant a biopsy because of the shape and size of the grouping of calcifications.

At this point I started to get a little worried because the last time I had a biopsy it came back positive for cancer. But I wasn't going to let myself get worked up until I had the procedure done and had the results in hand. And, if it was cancer again, I would beat this one too.

MARCH 19, 2020

Biopsy day. I had had biopsies before, so I thought I kind of knew what to expect. Boy, was I wrong. I lay on a cold hard table with my breasts hanging in a hole. Talk about letting ALL of your modesty go. The numbing process went smoothly, I hardly felt a thing, and luckily the same went for the actual biopsy. Just a little pressure and tugging. Three areas were biopsied and then the wait began. I should get my results within three to five days. Needless to say, I didn't get much sleep the days following the biopsy. A few days later, the results were back. NOT MALIGNANT, whoo-hoo! However, I wasn't out of the woods yet. The results came back as atypical epithelial hyperplasia, which is a precursor to cancer.

My surgeon wanted to go in again and take thicker margins with an excisional biopsy, to remove more tissue to ensure all the bad cells were gone. Okay, no problem, I need to do this.

During the same time, the dreaded COVID virus hit the US. Hospitals weren't performing any non-emergency procedures, so I had to wait to schedule my biopsy.

Fast forward almost three months. Hospitals are open again. Obviously, this whole time my diagnosis was on my mind. I was so relieved to finally be able to get an appointment and get this taken care of and over with.

JUNE 4, 2020

Today is my excisional biopsy day. Out of the three suspicious areas, two of them were close enough together to be biopsied with one incision. My surgeon wasn't sure this would be the case until she got inside and saw the areas. Wires were placed, and a mammogram was taken so she knew exactly where to incise since the areas were microscopic. The surgery went well, the two areas were biopsied, and I was sent home to wait on results.

My surgeon said if nothing was wrong, I would receive a call from her medical assistant, but if the results came back positive, she would call me herself. Jokingly she said, you DO

NOT want me to call you. We had a good laugh since this was basically just a precaution—or so we thought.

JUNE 8, 2020

It had been a long day at work, and I was done late. While driving home, I received a call from my surgeon's office. I answered it and when I heard my surgeon's voice, the tears immediately started to well up in my eyes. I remember saying, "Oooooh noooo," and her response was, "I'm so sorry I am the one calling you."

The first question I asked her was if I was dying. She replied with a firm no, but this was something to be taken seriously. Two different types of cancer had been found, two of the areas were HER2+ cancer, and there was an area of Invasive Ductal Carcinoma (IDC) they didn't even know was there until the bigger margins were taken and processed.

Wow, I had *cancer* . . . again. We talked for what seemed a very long time; I don't even remember driving the rest of the way home. I knew I had to tell my boyfriend, family, and friends. They would be worried, and I didn't want that for them. I wasn't going to let this get the better of me. I had to fight as hard as I could.

I was referred to an oncologist I would meet in the upcoming week. So surreal . . . I have an oncologist. The day I met him I could tell immediately I was in great hands. I was going to be okay. He was very knowledgeable, very compassionate, and very detailed.

My oncologist suggested I get genetic testing done, since breast cancer runs in my family, and because of my prior cancer history. Luckily, after all the blood work and visits my results came back negative for any abnormalities. He thought for sure my results would be positive, so this was a great surprise for both of us. Finally, a piece of good news.

I was given a few options for how we were going to go about treating my cancer. Chemo was definitely in my near future, as well as surgery. We just didn't know what type yet since they wanted to do a breast MRI of both sides to confirm the areas and see if anything new had appeared.

When I heard the word chemo, the first thing I asked is if I would lose my hair. That was really my main concern; after all, my hair was down to my lower back, and it was one of the things I was very proud of. He told me yes, I would lose all my hair, about two to three weeks after I started chemo. I started to cry, then apologized for being vain. He told me it was the number one question he was asked, since sometimes our hair is what defines us as women and to never apologize. Hair grows back. I knew I had to get healthy and chemotherapy was hopefully going to be the answer.

JUNE 19, 2020

Today was bilateral MRI day. Talk about claustrophobic. Face down, again. On a hard table, again. With my breasts in a hole, again. Done. Okay, let's hope this turns out positive. I really wanted to get the treatment started right away.

A few days later, my results were in. The left breast confirmed the suspicious masses and a lymph node in my left armpit looked bigger than normal. The right breast also had a suspicious looking mass they didn't see before. Oh, my goodness, what was happening?

Chemo was scheduled to begin in July, but they had to figure what drug and dosage was going to be administered since they kept finding new abnormalities. Both of my surgeons thought an ultrasound guided biopsy of all three areas would be best in determining the type of chemotherapy I would receive and the type of surgery I would have after my chemotherapy was complete.

Since I would be getting many infusions, my oncologist suggested I get a chemo port placed instead of having to inject the drugs in my arm every time. At this point, I was going to do whatever he suggested.

By this time, I had already had lengthy conversations with my employer about what was happening and the fact I would be having to take a long medical leave of absence since my immune system would be compromised and COVID-19 was in full effect. Typically, you can work through chemotherapy treatments, but not during a pandemic. The end of June would be my last day at my job of twelve years.

JULY 1, 2020

At my follow up appointment, my oncologist and I discussed my biopsy results a little further and he thought I would benefit by joining a clinical trial for my HER2 + breast cancer. With the research being done, they would be able to help other patients with my similar diagnosis. I had to think about it for a few days, but ultimately decided it would be a good thing to do. The only scary part was being randomized into a treatment category. Although I wasn't put into the group who would be receiving the new chemo drug, I was put into the standard-of-care group and I was happy about that.

Originally my treatment was going to be six chemo infusions: once every three weeks, along with two immunotherapy drugs. With the clinical trial, I was going to be receiving chemo once a week for twelve weeks, and every third week an infusion of Perjeta and Herceptin. The two immunotherapy drugs would help my own immune system fight the cancer. These infusions would be every three weeks for a year.

I was on board and ready to go. Let's get this started.

JULY 2, 2020

Today was my chemo port placement day. I'd had a handful of surgeries before, so this would be no big deal. The port was placed in my right upper chest and a catheter was threaded through a vein in my neck down into my vena cava above my heart. Today was the day it all became real for me. Now, I was officially ready to go.

JULY 3, 2020

For my bilateral ultrasound-guided biopsies, I had wires placed again, and another mammogram to make sure the correct areas were prepared. The biopsy sites were identified. Left breast, left armpit lymph node, and right breast new suspicious area. Luckily, I felt nothing, and all went well. By this time, I was a pro.

JULY 8, 2020

The results from the biopsies came back. The cancer had spread to my lymph nodes under my arm, but the mass in the right breast was benign. Having cancer in one breast is bad enough; thank goodness it wasn't both. More good news. I also got the news I was approved for the clinical trial and I would be starting chemotherapy the following week. I was so ready to be done with tests and to just begin my treatment.

Since I knew I was going to lose my hair, I made an appointment that weekend to get it cut super short to donate to a charity. I cried, but then realized I didn't look so bad with short hair, it was kind of fun. Too bad it was going to all fall out.

Thus far during my journey I had so many people reach out to me with positive thoughts, prayers, and advice. One of my friends told me about this wonderful lady named Deb who ran a nonprofit retreat for cancer survivors. Since I hadn't even started treatment yet, I didn't know what to expect when I contacted her, but to my surprise she suggested we do a chemo sendoff party on her river boat. I got to invite my friends and family and we spent a few hours on the river talking, laughing, eating, and just having fun before my upcoming journey. It really was a blessing and it meant so much to me. I am excited to do an actual retreat after I beat this cancer. Thank you, Deb, your kindness and strength are an inspiration.

JULY 15, 2020

Today was the first day of my twelve-week chemo and immunotherapy journey. Boy, was I anxious, scared, and excited to get it started. Since they didn't know how I would react to any of the drugs being administered the day was very long and tiring. Nine hours, in fact. I had to get my loading doses and the nurses monitored me very closely to make sure I had no side effects, which I didn't. The infusions went very well, better than I was expecting. No problems to report. I was hoping this would be the case the whole time. The next day I woke up and I felt great, even went for a few miles walk with some girlfriends. WOW, I thought, this is great. Boy, was I in for a rude awakening. The next day I could barely get out of bed, I was so tired. My skin had also developed a weird bumpy rash, but thankfully it went away in two days and never reappeared throughout the rest of the twelve weeks. That loading dose was no joke. Or it could have been the steroids I got as a premedication before every infusion.

As the weeks went on, and the infusions became a part of my weekly routine, the fatigue really began to kick in, especially after the weeks where I would receive all three drugs. I would inevitably be in bed for two days afterwards. I also received Benadryl as a premedication, which contributed to the sleepiness, but the chemotherapy was the major culprit.

By week three, sure enough, my hair started to slowly fall out. Every time I would run my fingers through it, I would come away with a handful of hair. I took a shower one day, and the amount of hair that fell out was astonishing. It literally happened overnight. I was in shock, but I knew it was going to happen, so I told myself to pull it together, it will grow back. As the days went on, with every shower, more and more hair fell out . . . in handfuls. By the third day of "hairmageddon," I asked my boyfriend to just shave the remaining hair off. I video messaged my mom and sister, and we had a good laugh-and-cry session as we said goodbye to my hair. Thankfully, to my surprise, my bald head didn't look too bad.

The only other side effects I had the whole time were some pretty harsh intestinal issues, brought on by the chemo and Perjeta (immunotherapy drug). Luckily, I was able to somewhat control it. It's still a bit of an issue but should go away once I stop all of my infusions. I cannot wait for that day. I feel like I was pretty lucky. I never got sick, I didn't feel sick, despite the fact I had aggressive Stage II cancer. With all I was going through, my oncologist kept telling me how lucky I was, since it was a fluke that I even had a mammogram in the first place. I agree with him.

Towards the end of my chemotherapy treatments, I had several appointments with my general surgeon and plastic surgeon to discuss my surgery options. One of the options was to have a double mastectomy with reconstruction, and the other was to have a lumpectomy and bilateral reduction and lift. From the beginning of this ordeal, breast conservation was the opinion and goal of both surgeons. The risks, pros, and cons were given to me for both options and now I had a decision to make. My first thought was to go for the double mastectomy. Just get both breasts removed, have reconstruction, end of story. My surgeon and oncologist told me to think hard about it because reconstruction wasn't always what people thought it would be. I also found out that I would have to have radiation after my surgery since the cancer had spread to my lymph nodes. Decisions, decisions.

SEPTEMBER 29, 2020

MY LAST CHEMO INFUSION. I can't believe how quickly those twelve weeks went. Now I had a break for a month to get my immune system back to normal before my surgery. I also had to make a surgical decision. Time was moving fast.

OCTOBER 9, 2020

I had a follow up MRI today to see if the chemo had done its job. Sure enough, all the masses and the lymph nodes had shrunk and were back to normal size. There were no other signs of abnormalities. The chemo worked. Thank goodness. Since everything had shrunk, the best surgical option for me would be to save my breasts, but because of the size of the areas where the cancer was, I was told my plastic surgeon would have to be creative at the time of removal and reconstruction. I was ready.

OCTOBER 14, 2020

I met my radiation oncologist today. Since radiation was necessary with either surgical path, I knew I had made the right decision. She was pretty positive the radiation would be the best thing for me for preventing a recurrence of cancer. Radiation would consist of five weeks of treatments, Monday through Friday. The treatments would start after my surgery.

OCTOBER 28, 2020

Surgery day. For most of my adult life I had always wanted to get a breast reduction, this just wasn't how I wanted to have it happen, but there is always a silver lining when it's free! My surgery, a partial mastectomy of the left breast, bilateral reduction and lift, and the removal of six lymph nodes in my left armpit, was about five hours long. Because of COVID, I wasn't allowed to have anyone in the room with me, so I woke up alone.

I was told the surgery went very well, and I had wonderful new boobs. I stayed one night in the hospital, with no pain throughout the night or the next morning. My plastic surgeon came by the next day to check on me and I got to see my new breasts for the first time. I was very pleased; he had done an exceptional job. They were perfect. The only downfall was I had two drains, one in each breast. I had to take care of the drains and empty them three times a day for the next week. It wasn't as bad as I thought. I had very little pain. I wasn't allowed to lift my arms or lift anything heavy for a week. I healed very well. After a week I had the stitches and drains removed, and my surgeon said I was healing ahead of schedule. I'll take it.

Once again, my body had to heal. After about three weeks,

I was almost back to normal, with no pain at all. Some soreness and twinges is all I experienced. I felt very lucky. What an experience this has been so far.

NOVEMBER 6, 2020

Surgery results were back, and I had no more cancer in my body. I could finally take a deep breath. There was a light at the end of this very dark tunnel I was in.

DECEMBER 15, 2020

My first day of radiation. Because the area to be irradiated was close to my heart and lungs, I would have to do what is called the hold breath technique while the radiation was being administered. The hold breath technique entails your nose being plugged, and breathing through a snorkel, until the time of radiation, then you take two breaths and one deep breath and hold it for about 20–30 seconds. This would be my life for the next five weeks. The first day I was very nervous because I didn't know if I could hold my breath for that long. Multiple times during each treatment. It was easier than I thought. It took them longer to set me up than the actual time the treatment took.

So far, I have a little swelling, some redness, and some fatigue, but no significant side effects. I will take this as a blessing in disguise.

I have been very fortunate in all of my treatment and I am so thankful I made the decision to go and get a mammogram. It was probably my best decision yet. I have so much life ahead of me and I can't wait to be done and healthy again.

Much love and peace!

Lauren Oman

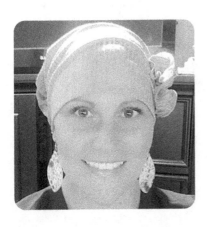

Lauren Oman has worked as a dental assistant for nineteen years, a job she loves.

Lauren and her boyfriend Matt enjoy the outdoors; fishing, clamming, crabbing, going to the beach, and spending time on their boat. She also loves dogs and enjoys quilting and painting.

It was June 2020 when they diagnosed Lauren with Stage II HER2 Positive Invasive Ductal Carcinoma. Cancer had also spread to the lymph nodes in her left arm.

Lauren went through twelve consecutive weeks of chemotherapy. She had a partial mastectomy of the left breast with bi-lateral reconstruction, and twenty-five rounds of radiation. She is about to complete a year of immunotherapy infusions.

Lauren had no symptoms at her very first mammogram when she received a diagnosis of breast cancer. Because of this, she advocates and encourages women to have their mammograms.

Support from family and friends made her journey bearable.

Connect with Lauren
Email: Honeygirl10@hotmail.com
Instagram: @frogger12345
Website: https://laurenoman.po.sh

The best things in life aren't things

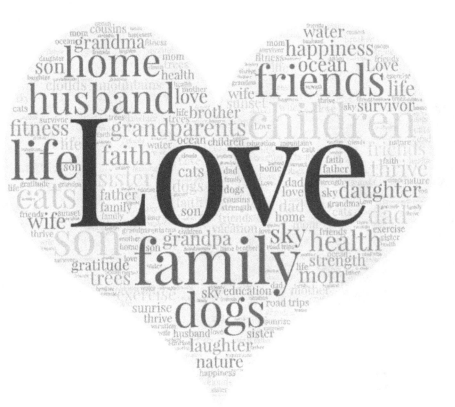

CHAPTER FIVE
IT HAPPENED TO ME
ROBYN MCMANAMA

I SOMETIMES CANNOT BELIEVE it happened to me. I was the one on the receiving end of a phone call hearing "you have cancer." It felt like time stood still, and just for a moment I was on the outside watching this happen to someone else. And then it hit me —it was me; I was the one with cancer.

I was only thirty-five at the time I was diagnosed. Too young for regular mammograms. I was in for my annual exam with my nurse midwife when she felt a lump in each of my breasts. She thought they were cysts but sent me in for a mammogram anyway.

Afterwards, multiple doctors said her gut instinct had saved my life. The biopsy determined a couple days later I had Stage II Invasive Ductal Carcinoma (IDC) in my right breast, and it was growing at an 80% proliferation rate. (This is how quickly a cancer cell copies its DNA and divides into two cells. The higher the number, the more aggressive it is.) The lump in my left breast was benign. I remember being on the phone with the doctor who had done my biopsy, thinking I literally had no idea what to do now. Was I supposed to call someone or go somewhere? My mind was racing but felt completely blank at the same time. Thankfully, the doctor told me she would get things started and she referred me to two different breast surgeons and within a couple hours both offices had reached out to schedule an appointment.

From that point on, everything was a whirlwind. After I decided on a surgical oncologist, it was port surgery, chemo class, pick up meds, tell people, research side effects. In the middle of this, my husband Ryan and I had to figure out how to tell our two daughters their mom had breast cancer and life was going to change drastically. Our daughters were seven and ten at the time. We never wanted them to feel left out or not a part of what was happening so we were very honest with them about my illness and how chemo would make me sick. Our younger daughter didn't fully understand what it all meant but our older one did, and she took it hard, but we stressed we would get through this if we all supported each other.

Our friends and family did not miss a beat and we were immediately wrapped with prayer, messages, meals, childcare, and anything else we could think of. No one should have to walk a cancer diagnosis alone and we were so grateful for our community and how they carried us when it was too hard for us to move on our own.

CHEMOTHERAPY

About two weeks after my diagnosis, I had my first round of chemotherapy. The cancer was characterized as triple positive (ER/PR/HER2+) so I was given TCHP (Taxol, Carboplatin, Herceptin and Perjeta). I was prescribed six rounds of chemo, given every three weeks. All things considered, I handled the first and second rounds of chemo well. I was fatigued, nauseous, and my mouth lost all its tastebuds, but I was not overly sick. I had heard horror stories of how sick other patients had become from chemo, so I was very thankful.

One memory that will always be special for our family was the day I decided it was time to shave my hair. It had begun falling out in clumps exactly two weeks after my first treatment and I knew I needed to take control of it rather than feel pain and loss every time I saw my hands full of hair. My husband and daughters took turns cutting my hair short and then finally shaving it. We laughed and cried together, and my girls and I spent time trying on the different head coverings I had bought. In the end, the act of shaving my head was difficult but also empowering. My bald head was a symbol of what I was going through, and I wore it proudly.

Then things got a little rough after my third round of chemo. I thought I was doing well—it was spring break, and we took our daughters to a Broadway show and then had plans to head up to our family's vacation home at Mt. Hood. However, after the show my heart just didn't feel right. It was beating too quickly and irregularly. I was advised to head to the closest ER, and I was admitted just minutes after arriving. They did a battery of tests but were unable to diagnose what was going on. However, because I was currently going through chemo-therapy, they decided to keep me for observation. Over the next couple of days, I was put through every heart and stress test they could think of. The only conclusion was I was having a bad reaction to the Neulasta shot (to keep my white blood cell count from dropping) I received after each chemo, and they put me on beta blockers. This seemed to do the trick and I was able to complete my last three rounds of chemo without any incident.

TIME FOR SURGERY

One (of many) things I've learned is there are many types of breast cancer and along with that, many different treatment plans. My triple positive cancer was one of the most aggressive, which means chemo first with the goal of stopping it from spreading while also trying to shrink the tumors before surgery. One of the benefits of this was the extra time it gave me to research and decide what kind of surgery I would have (lumpectomy vs. mastectomy). I had also learned at the beginning of this journey I was positive for a genetic mutation called RAD50. This gives me a higher predisposition for both breast and ovarian cancer. Because of this, my doctors and I decided on a bilateral mastectomy for my surgery. I had my last round of chemotherapy at the end of May and I was given a few weeks to rest and recover before surgery which thankfully lined up with a family trip to Hawaii. What a wonderful time it was! We celebrated, rested, and tried our best to leave our cancer cares back home.

My mastectomy surgery and recovery went well. My husband was my rock—he tracked my pain medications, made sure I ate, helped me move around, and charted my drain output. (Now that's true love!) At the time of my mastectomy, it was not known if I would need radiation, so my reconstruction was delayed, and I was given expanders in the meantime. If you want to know what it feels like to have breast expanders, just imagine two rocks strapped to your chest. They are hard and uncomfortable but have an important job to do. Unfortunately, about four months after the mastectomy, one of my expanders became infected. I got extremely sick and ended up in the hospital for three days before they decided to remove the expander, clean out the area and replace it with a new one.

Thankfully it worked and I had no other issues with the expanders.

The findings after the mastectomy were that the cancer had not spread to my lymph nodes, so radiation was not needed. However, I did have residual cancer left (the goal is a 100% response rate) so I was prescribed to start a new kind of chemotherapy called Kadcyla. The typical regimen for Kadcyla is an infusion every three weeks for fourteen rounds. After my third round of Kadcyla, my eyes had an allergic reaction and it caused me to begin to lose my eyesight. Thankfully this was caught quickly, and I was taken off of Kadcyla and put back on the previously prescribed regimen of Herceptin and Perjeta (targeted therapy) for a year.

In between my mastectomy and delayed reconstruction, I had a total hysterectomy. This was done prophylactically due to the genetic mutation. It has been a struggle to go into surgical menopause overnight at the age of thirty-six. The menopause symptoms started up almost immediately, but I have been working with a naturopath who has me on supplements to help combat the symptoms which has helped a lot.

After a ton of research, I opted for a DIEP (deep inferior epigastric perforators) Flap reconstruction. This is a microvascular surgery that uses lower abdominal tissue, skin, and fat as the donor tissue (instead of implants). It is a ten-to-twelve-hour surgery and requires a night in the ICU for careful monitoring and then several more nights on the surgical recovery floor. Reconstruction is a very personal decision and after a lot of careful thought and conversations I decided this was what was best for me.

I was scheduled to have my DIEP Flap in March 2020, just a few weeks after the world started to shut down due to COVID-19. As hospitals began to cancel non-emergency surgeries, I learned mine too had been canceled. I understood why but I was devastated. This surgery was meant to mark the end of the biggest part of my cancer journey and I was anxious to have it completed. Also, I was desperate to have those expanders removed!

Since I was one of the first surgeries to be cancelled, I was lucky to later be one of the first ones to be rescheduled. In August I had my long-awaited DIEP Flap reconstruction surgery. It took twelve hours in total and went off without a hitch. The first night in the ICU was rough, as the nurse had to check the flaps every thirty minutes, not giving me much opportunity for sleep. Thankfully, this only lasted for the first twenty-four hours, and then the frequency of checks decreased to every hour for another twenty-four hours, and then eventually every couple of hours.

The hard part about this type of reconstruction is that it involves two major surgical sites. I was unable to use my arms to move myself around and had lost all use of my abdominal muscles as well. The next day, I learned quickly that the daytime ICU nurse was no-nonsense and was determined to show me I was still able to move on my own. She helped me out of bed for the first time since surgery and got me sitting in a chair. When it came time to transfer me out of the ICU into a patient recovery room and the patient transporter arrived with the wheelchair, the nurse would not allow me to sit in it—she insisted I walk! So, walk I did, all the way to my new room, across the entire hospital, from one end to the other. Not only did she show me I was able to walk that far, but I became famous for it! Over the next three days, every nurse who came in my room said they had heard about how I walked all the way from the ICU.

My last surgery was four months after the first part of the

reconstruction. DIEP Flap is a multistep process, with at least two revisions. By this time, I was experiencing major surgery fatigue. It is hard to stop life for a surgery and spend weeks healing only to start over. I asked my plastic surgeon if there was any way he could combine the two revisions—which he agreed to do. It made for a longer surgery and a tougher recovery but I'm very thankful to say that after two years of surgeries and treatments, there are no more on the horizon!

For now, I will continue taking an aromatase inhibitor for the next five to seven years and will receive an infusion of Zometa every six months. These medications work to keep my bones strong, both to resist recurrence and to prevent osteoporosis from setting in.

EXERCISING THROUGH TREATMENT

I have always been an athlete, and exercise has long been a part of my daily routine. In the beginning I committed to myself that if I couldn't do anything else, I would at least go for a walk *every single day*. And walk I did. Some days I could only make it to the mailbox and back, but as I regained my strength after each procedure, my walks lengthened. When I was strong enough, I would work my way back to my normal exercise routines. I'm so thankful that for the most part I recovered from my treatments and surgeries quickly. I attribute it to the fact that every day, if I couldn't do anything else, I at least got up and out for a short walk.

On the day of my diagnosis, my younger brother committed to me that as soon as I was healthy, we would complete a half Ironman together (something that had long been on my bucket list). I am now registered for a race later this year in Arizona and am officially training! It will be a huge goal completion; I can't wait to have my family there cheering me on. I'm excited to do something after cancer I've never done before—to prove that not only is cancer not going to defeat me but that I will come back stronger than ever!

PINK SISTAS

I first learned about Pink Sistas from a couple girlfriends who had attended a retreat with Deb Hart. I connected with Deb and expressed interest in attending a retreat as well. Sadly, it has yet to happen because all social activities were suspended due to COVID-19. However, Deb has followed my story on social media and has always been very supportive and encouraging. I'm thankful to have connected with her and I look forward to being able to attend a retreat in the future!

WHAT COMES NEXT

I think all cancer survivors know cancer is never "over" in the true sense of the word. Yes, active treatment and surgeries have ended. Yes, I've been declared NED (no evidence of disease) . . . thank you, Jesus! But cancer will always be a nagging thought in the back of my mind. Does that new pain mean the cancer has metastasized? It will always be my reality that I could face a recurrence. And I will always be dealing with the long-term effects from the treatments and surgeries.

I am grateful for every day I get to wake up and be a wife and mom. I'm thankful I get to continue to watch my girls grow older. I'm grateful for how cancer pulled us closer together as a family. I'm grateful for the women I've met along the way, each with their own unique story that has bonded us into a tribe of warriors.

She is clothed in dignity and strength and can laugh without fear of the future.

PROVERBS 31:25

Robyn McManama

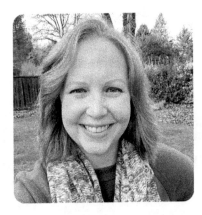

Robyn McManama is a native Californian, but she has called Oregon her home for the past twenty years.

For ten years she owned and operated two resale clothing stores until she chose to stay home full-time with her daughters while they were young.

Robyn, her husband Ryan, and daughters Lilly and Samantha have an active lifestyle of bike riding, hiking, traveling, and adventuring together. She works part time at her daughters' school, helping to tutor children and substitute where needed.

Exercise has always been a priority and passion for Robyn. When she received her breast cancer diagnosis, she set her sights on completing a Half Ironman once she finished treatment. She is now enjoying training for her race, volunteering, and living a life that doesn't revolve so much around her diagnosis.

Robyn loves Jesus, her family, and her friends. She is grateful to wake up each morning and live out her life as fully as possible, knowing each day is a gift.

Connect with Robyn
Email: rlmcmanama@gmail.com
Facebook: Robyn McManama
Instagram: @70.3aftercancer
(Follow her journey to complete her first Half Ironman)

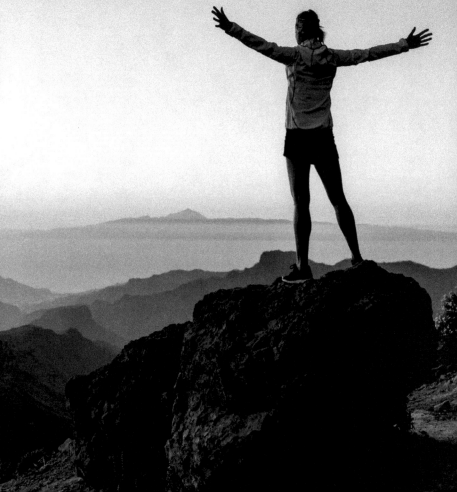

CHAPTER SIX
CHAMPIONS NEEDED
SHERRIDA PRECIADO GATES

You ARE MY ADVOCATE. Mine, and many others who have traveled this path. You bought a copy of this collection of epic stories. You are either a survivor, a supporter, a philanthropist, or curious. Either way, you have lifted our voices with your contribution. I thank you for your persistence.

Each of us has a story. It could be sad, scary, frightful, treacherous, happy, ecstatic, or just true to you and me. A single line or crack in an individual life. We embody our birth, fears, pain, successes, death, and rebirth. We must really incorporate so much into one person and one lifetime; we will need to share the wealth. I guess it is what I intend to do. For each of you who read this will believe it to be some sort of tribute or a cautionary tale. I hope to leave a mark on you. My intentions are good and fair, not malicious or threatening. For as I speak my history you too could be bound to repeat it to others for their good, and so on, as the game of gossip goes.

So many tales and traditions are handed down by women throughout this world—whether at a quilting bee, the wash pool, over the fences, or the harvesting fields where they exchange their experiences of pain and suffering, women carry that burden and honor. Does it all make me sound dated and out of touch? More and more of us are rising up to meet the challenges as we use Facebook, Twitter, our neighborhood watch, schools, and church websites accordingly. If we continue to voice our histories out loud and in public, in time we would warrant actions and results. We are all mature and discrete enough to decide what bears repeating.

If we remain silent and composed over our endangered health, why would anyone respond and fight for us. All of us have heard this before and we all want it to be true. It starts with this and many hundreds of other stories that will educate our daughters, sisters, aunts, and all the women who will come to be. This is the twenty-first century and you would think I was talking of something that happened quite a long time ago when women had very few rights and privileges. We have all heard the time-honored saying, "Don't wash your dirty laundry in public." This goes beyond that.

Please let me enlighten you on the ever so present cause for women and the rights of their own choices for their bodily health. Breast cancer was initially a taboo conversation and it was individual activism and supportive groups that increased its research/education.

While it remained a hidden disease, the funding for cancer research and education was little more than what was used to fund an advertisement for toothpaste. With the help of the right people in the right places, the words "breast cancer" and its devastating toll was starting to come into the light. Other women of means and fame, upon dealing with the cavalier attitudes of their doctors who quickly performed mastectomies and never bothered to answer a single question on what other options might be available or what was next for the women post-breast cancer, fought for help and education. Our sister's efforts to develop and fund research, recovery support groups and counseling has been to our advantage. Today we are able to benefit from their unselfish actions, and we must continue to pay it forward.

Like some women, I knew very little of my mom's side of the family's health history and even less of the other side. I believe what held me together and urged me to work harder for a more positive outcome with my cancer was my intent of giving good history and facts to my daughter. I was not going to allow my children to be swimming in the dark waters that can engulf you during a health crisis not of their making.

I felt way too young for a diagnosis of cancer. I was forty-five, almost forty-six. I had a daughter just starting high school and an even younger son. Monica and Jonah are everything to me. I had left my career to raise them and continue to do all I can to be present for their life experiences. Craig, my husband of twenty-one years at the time of diagnosis, was moving along in his career and life was just your basic bliss. We have traveled and lived overseas in Ireland for a few years and have been very lucky to visit a lot of countries. We had both been in the military after college and stationed around the States. Our lifestyle choices had been much influenced by this travel, as well as our own decisions to be healthier and fitter than our families.

While Craig had a history of growing up without a variety of food options, I was raised by a mother who was a good cook for the times. My mom's family had bouts when each of them were overweight and Craig's family also had some poor eating habits. We ate a little differently and chose to eat local. I baked our bread and grew a lot of our produce. We were in sports, activities, church, volunteering, classes, and we hosted exchange students for many years. We stayed active and healthy in comparison to our familial history. Once I was diagnosed, the researching and changes began. I no longer "kick" myself over my apparently decent choices. Maybe too much Guinness while living in Ireland, or too much sugar visiting other countries? Or maybe I wasn't responsible for my breast cancer. Life is uncertain.

JUST MISSED IT

In the early years after our return to the States, we were all connected back to our preferred primary doctors and dentists. I got the kids all their school physicals, while in the meantime noticing how tired I was. I mentioned it in passing to my primary doctor; he blew it off. I did not take it rudely, but just figured he knew best, and I was just fine. I guess I just took for granted or maybe burdened him to be able to look at me and know all there is to know, medically speaking, that is. For the next two to three years, I made a number of appointments looking for an answer to why I was always tired. It was never even a blip on the radar what might be going on.

In the years leading up to my diagnosis I lost a brother to suicide, another brother and his family were having devastating difficulties, and the job security at my husband's company was shaky.

My doctor gave me a plethora of choices for my state of health. I was told how I was aging, having a busy life with very active children, I could expect to see a little drop in my energy once in a while. These answers were fine for a portion of the time. Now, I look at everything through different lenses. I truly had few health issues and never needed to be worried or ask for more. Didn't even think I had the right to ask for anything. The old adage about the "customer always being right" never seems to fit in the medical office. No one ever asked for blood work or had me on anything other than patronizing responses. I started to get frustrated. I was not sleeping well, gaining weight, depressed, and pain-free, but I had some anxiety. Apparently, you can feel this way and your doctor will bless you with how well you are coping with motherhood.

I had my first mammogram at forty-five, almost forty-six. They saw nothing out of the ordinary. Good. I didn't expect anything irregular. I was scheduled to get my son in for some shots before school started at our primary care facility.

All was going well; they were late, but it was usually the case these days. I needed to know how much longer, as he and I were getting cranky. When we finally got in, after the shots, my doctor asked my son to wait outside the door while he spoke to me. He let me know he had just been placed in charge of the facility and wanted to know how I felt about the service. I felt a little rewarded because he wanted my opinion. Lucky me. I was honest but curtailed. "Well, it was fine. I felt it had gotten a little harder to make appointments and get seen on time recently." He thanked me and then promptly let me know I needed to find a better suited facility as I seemed rather frustrated at times with him. I had been "fired."

I literally broke down and cried. In hindsight, he had not been able to find what was wrong with me, so "I" was the problem. I had continued to express doubt in his diagnosis therefore "I" needed to leave. I was awestruck. It's hard to find primary care doctors in the area and I was being cast out without a net of hope to reel me back in. It was like a bad breakup. You know what they say about those types of relationships? Incredible changes are about to happen. Now I needed to take better control of what I had power over.

SHAKE MYSELF AWAKE

Over the past twelve years and more during my treatment, I questioned and researched how to "not do" or "not eat" or "not think." I truly believe information-seeking was my coping measure. In gathering the most up-to-date information, I can regain control and understand my situation and deal with the topics that arise.

I have volunteered with support programs who have put on educational seminars and spoken myself; done conferences, runs, walks, fashion shows, fly fishing, auctions, intimacy courses, cooking classes, make-up aid, massages, journaling, yoga, dietitians, and partook in all that assisted cancer survivors. I found my family was learning from me and my experience. My own friends and community started to ask me for information, or at least direction.

Early on, my parents and in-laws could not really see the treatment or the support as anything more than prolonging the inevitable. I believe they became a little more enlightened with our choices. My journey was quite arduous and very scary. After being set adrift by my longtime primary care group, I just paused for a bit. Other things were going on and I was getting back into the work field, it just was too much to handle for the times. The rest of the family was still welcome at the clinic, just not me. I made an appointment with my gynecologist for the annual. I told her how I felt and asked her about the weight gain under the arm. At first, I got the same little "oh, you're getting older and hormones are changing to create fatty areas around your body." Now, I am petite, 5'2", and I have stayed pretty much in shape. I was in the military, knew I had to keep taking care of myself, and was determined to do so. I asked her about scheduling some way to look into the area better. It wasn't symmetrical. After it came back noted "area of concern," then we got the ball rolling. It was diagnosed as Triple Positive (ER, HER2, and PR) Ductal carcinoma in situ (DCIS), Stage IIB. The HER2 protein positivity attracted the most attention from the medical professionals. The tumor was quite large and aggressive. After surgery had established cancer had not spread to my lymphatic system, I was directed towards my treatment plan. As we do not live anywhere near either of our families, my best friend and husband set up fantastic support from everywhere. Church, work, and community all came in on the proverbial white horses, granting my every spoken need and unspoken wishes.

ADORN MY CAPE

As the signs of my adapting to the breast cancer diagnosis started to appear Craig was working to provide the practical support, which helped in maintaining my self-confidence. He is, after all, a chemical engineer. The depression and anxiety that often set in were clear signs I did not feel in control. My life had drastically changed. I was going through three years plus of aggressive chemotherapy, radiation therapy, infusions for HER2+, more surgery, and aromatase inhibitors.

My side effects were all over the map. I was thrown cruelly into post-menopause and am still receiving those gifts. Even today, I still have uncomfortable CIPN (chemo-induced peripheral neuropathy), osteopenia, continued cognitive challenges, and your run-of-the-mill intimacy struggles. My journey was similar in many ways to others around me, but I really would not have been aware of them without the support of many programs, delivered unselfishly. You see, those who advocated for changes, empowerment, and no more silence about breast cancer are the true heroes. They were there to ask: How does one deal with the guilt of putting your children through this? Navigate the negative tendencies into positive thinking. The managing of distress, balancing work and cancer, and simply not wallowing in self-hate and pity. The feelings of complete and utter inadequacy in your relationship. "My body —my goodness, what is happening?" These were all a part of the forever journey I continue on.

The programs that are worth your money, energy, and promotion, are the ones in which cancer survivors bare their souls or not. Retreats like the ones put on by Pink Sistas in Portland, Oregon. They allow you to come, in peace, to accept yourself for where you are and be loved by a sisterhood you now belong to. It is how one moves on. Moving on is not a direction per se, more of an acknowledgment. Most cancer survivors like to know where they are, where they have been, and a little insight into where they might be headed. One advocates for oneself by choosing a direction. An informed and supported path and speaking up about it never hurts either.

You know I just wanted to follow up on the primary care doctor who fired me. I'd like to say he sent me cards and flowers, reporting he had changed his ways and was truly sorry, but you know better. What did occur was I was out having coffee with a friend and bumped into him. I said hello and asked if he remembered me—it had been four years. He replied yes and asked how I was doing. I exclaimed how he had saved my life. I graciously thanked him for his due diligence in kicking me out of his practice four years before. I went on to explain, and yes, calmly. I had survived breast cancer and had he not pushed me to look elsewhere for a better, more thorough physician, I might not be standing here in front of him today. He had a wide-eyed look of "oh, crap." I said in a very kind and professional voice, "Maybe in the future, when a female patient is telling you she is not feeling well and her body, in which she has lived for a long time and knows well, is telling her something is wrong, you might listen and take her for her word and try harder." He gave a slight smile of acknowledgment and we said our goodbyes. What may be most important is to never give up on getting an answer that allows peace, because most of us know when something isn't right.

Sherrida Preciado Gates

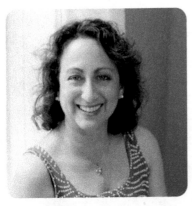

Sherri Gates grew up in a military family and moved often as a young girl.

She comes from a large family, and easily made friends, and quickly got involved wherever they were stationed.

She joined the United States Air Force after graduating college and working for several years in social work. She loved the military and the educational opportunities available to pursue. Sherri and her husband Craig met while they were both serving in the military.

Sherri and Craig have two children, Monica and Jonah. The family lived in Ireland for two years and loves to travel. The children were experts at packing and pulling their bags everywhere they visited.

Craig accepted a job in the Pacific Northwest after graduation, so Sherri finished her military obligation and they moved west.

Sherri loves her home, and although she can make a home anywhere, she is happy to stay where she is.

"Adventure always awaits!"

Connect with Sherri
Email: svgates8@gmail.com
Facebook: Sherri Gates

Everything
is just perspective

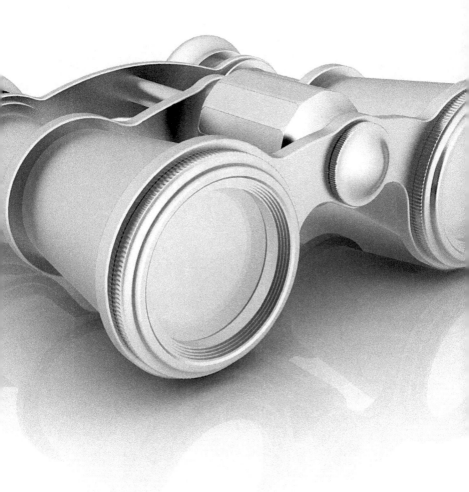

CHAPTER SEVEN
TREVA'S STORY
TREVA VETTER

CANCER HAS AFFECTED me since the day I was born. While my mom was pregnant with me, she didn't know it yet, but she had breast cancer. After I was born my mom had troubles with breast pain while breastfeeding me. Her pain was dismissed as mastitis and she was sent home. After all, she was only twenty-eight years old and doctors didn't believe she could have breast cancer at such a young age.

After many doctor's appointments, Mom was finally diagnosed with breast cancer. I was too young to remember her going through her first breast cancer treatment as I was only an infant but I was told she did have a unilateral mastectomy, chemotherapy, and radiation. Unfortunately, Mom learned a few years later that her treatment didn't work. To my parents' disappointment, the cancer returned, and Mom had to remove the other breast and continue with chemotherapy.

I do have a few memories of Mom. During her recurrence, she taught me how to blow wishes, and she taught me "he loves me, he loves me not" with daisies. I remember my mom being very ill with chemotherapy. I have one memory of her sitting down to brush my hair and then having to get up quickly and run to the bathroom to vomit in the toilet. She was really trying to be available to us, but the chemotherapy was taking a toll on her. I have a few other memories of my sister and me playing catch with her fake boobs in the house. She never told us girls to stop; she probably didn't have enough energy to muster up the words.

Mom also was desperately trying to break me from having a security blanket and sucking my thumb. I had a ratty old soft white blanket I carried around just like Linus from the Peanuts comic strip. She was so embarrassed of the blanket and worried I would suck my thumb forever. Grandma had knitted me a new blanket that was purple and pink, and I remember they tricked me and told me I could have the new blanket if I gave them my blanket. I reluctantly did the trade but immediately wanted my blanket back; sure enough, they wouldn't give it to me, and it was thrown out. I felt so deceived that she had tricked me into giving up my favorite blanket.

I have one other memory of Mom being so excited to watch a movie that was on television. We couldn't get the TV antenna to work in the living room, so she cozied up in her bedroom and watched "One Flew Over the Cuckoo's Nest" with me, with the tinfoil on a small black-and-white TV. I was bored with the movie, but it was something Mom really wanted to watch. The movie was filmed at the Oregon State Hospital right down the street from where I was born. She was thrilled a mainstream movie was filmed in our own backyard.

Mom was receiving treatment in Salem, Oregon, but since things were not going very well, she moved her treatment to Portland, Oregon. She would have to go to Portland and stay for a week at a time while my sister and I stayed with extended family. My family wouldn't speak of the cancer in front of me and my sister. At the time, I didn't even know Mom had cancer. I just thought she was sick. I could see her wearing wigs and throwing up, and she had fake boobs she wore in her bra, but I wasn't at an age where I could put two and two together.

There were lots of whispering conversations between the adults. All of this happened before I was in primary school. My mom taught me the alphabet and colors when she had time, getting me ready to join the big kids and prepared to enter first grade. My favorite toy they had bought me was a toy called "Light and Learn" from Sesame Street. I spent hours playing with that modern-day computer.

One evening my Dad took my sister and me to the hospital to see Mom. Apparently, we were not allowed in the room to see her. We were too young, the hospital had visitation rules and children were not allowed. Dad snuck us in for one quick hug and then we got shooed away and we waited patiently out in the hallway for Dad to finish his visit. I believe we stayed in Portland that night at our aunt's house.

The next day Dad returned to the hospital to be with Mom while my sister and I stayed behind at my aunt's house to play with my cousins. That evening when Dad returned, he sat my sister and me on the couch and got down on his knees to talk to us. My aunt stood behind the couch and I knew something wasn't right as Dad was shaking and Aunt Adeline was crying. Dad told us the news: Mom wasn't coming home, she had passed away. My sister started crying and my dad embraced her. I didn't cry, and Dad was frustrated as he didn't think I knew what he meant. He tried to find other words to tell me what had happened, but he didn't need to do that. I knew exactly what happened. I just couldn't talk, I couldn't cry, and I didn't know quite what to do. I sat there with a lump in my throat, but I didn't want to cry. I am not sure if I thought I was going to get in trouble for crying. My dad didn't tolerate listening to his girls cry very well, so I sat there in silence and told myself to be strong and not cry.

The ride home was a difficult two-hour commute. My sister took the front seat and I sat in the back of the Trailblazer by myself. We usually sat in the back together. We rode home in silence. No one spoke the entire time.

Soon after, we attended Mom's funeral. My sister and I were dressed in twin red velvet dresses with our hair done nicely and Dad wore a suit for the first time. The funeral was in Stayton, Oregon. I don't remember a word of the service, but I remember the open casket. My aunt picked me up and carried me to my mom to say one final good-bye. I was five years old. I don't know why I wasn't terrified, but again I told myself I was going to be strong.

I remember after the service Dad, my sister, and I got in the hearse and we were taken to the Gates Cemetery to lay Mom in her final resting place. I was so small I could stand up in the hearse and not even touch my head to the ceiling. It seemed a long drive; I suppose it was because I was only five years old and thirty-minute car rides seem like an eternity. At the cemetery, three chairs were placed at Mom's grave. They sat us down in order of age. Dad sat on the end, my sister sat in the middle, and I sat at the other end while our family gathered around behind us. We watched as they lowered Mom into the ground. Dad and my sister both cried while I sat there with the largest lump in my throat, holding back tears.

Growing up without a mom was different from anyone else that I knew. It was tough, but I got through it. As a child, my support system was very wide. I attended a small school where everyone was more like family. Whenever I wanted to go to a school function where I needed adult supervision, one of the school bus drivers would volunteer to be my guardian for the evening. I was a good kid, so they really didn't need to do anything! My neighbors ended up being my second family. I was over there often on the weekends and was there for all of our holiday celebrations.

I loved leaving a May Day basket on the porch for my neighbor Kelly. Kelly was the best mother a girl could have! Mother's Day was probably the toughest; in art class, the teacher would always have us make a gift to bring home to our moms. I would always balk at the idea but was told I needed to participate and to bring it home for my dad. Now that I am older, I don't know if it was such a good idea. I think bringing home something to Dad when it was meant for Mom probably would have been a pretty emotional thing for him.

We lived on a 120-acre cattle ranch and it always brought me more joy than misery. I loved the animals. We always had cows and horses. We occasionally had goats, sheep, or pigs. I even had one pet chicken! I loved that chicken. I caught the chicken at the Sisters Rodeo. My chicken slept with the dogs and really thought it was a dog. It would eat their food and fight with them just like a sibling.

Summers were the best growing up on the ranch. Every year we would harvest our hay and set it up in the barn so the animals would have enough food for the winter. Dad worked in the plywood mills. When he left for work, he would set me up to drive the tractor, and to cut, rake, and even bail the hay. On the weekend, his friends and their sons would be over, and we would work all weekend to take loads of hay into the barn.

My job was to drive the tractor or align the hay bales in a row so the hay elevator would pick up the hay more easily. The hay barn was always my solace. I would go out there every day after school to feed the cows, make hay forts, and swing from the rafters and jump into a soft pile of hay. I would spend hours out there by myself. Sometimes my sister would join me and take turns jumping. As we got older, she lost interest in spending time in the barn, but I still spent my time there feeding and talking to the animals.

The other amazing thing I loved about the ranch was the river that ran through the property. Our friends would come over every year and we would walk down to the river to go swimming. Each year the water eroded the banks of our land so our swimming holes changed from year to year. But each summer brought so much fun, whether it was swimming in the river, harvesting the garden, hauling in the hay, or making homemade ice cream and topping it with fresh blackberries, it all brought so much joy!

Dad ended up remarrying twice, once when I was ten; he was divorced by the time I was fourteen. My sister moved out when I was fifteen. Dad fell on tough times and often the bills were unpaid. We had no phone, and at times the electricity was turned off until the bill got paid. Dad was single, and sometimes he wouldn't come home for a week, so I occasionally would stay the night at my friend's house so I wouldn't be alone. A year later, at sixteen, I met an older man and starting dating. We married three years later when I was nineteen. At the time, I felt as if I was in love and had married the man of my dreams, but as I look back on the marriage it was done out of survival and the need for stability in my life. We never had children and divorced ten years later.

I worked my way through nursing school with the support of my husband, which gave me a great education to get me through this world. I started out as a Certified Nurse's Assistant and really enjoyed working in the nursing home. It was a great start to my nursing career. I then obtained my LPN and RN and transitioned to working in the local community hospital where I worked in acute care and critical care. After I divorced, I quit my job to start a journey with travel nursing. I wanted to see where the world could take me.

I plotted and planned my way to Long Island, New York, and took a position at North Shore Plainview Hospital for three months. The end of the three months couldn't come soon enough. I learned the hard way that when hospitals need travel nurses, they are in a staffing crisis. My first day on the job I had thirteen patients. It is just not a safe staffing ratio. I am not a quitter, though, I stayed on through my assignment but made it known I would not be picking up any extra shifts with the current staffing.

My apartment on Long Island was also something I had a really hard time acclimating to. Working night shift with the thin walls in the apartment was a challenge. I never slept well; I could even hear when the upstairs neighbor would walk across the apartment to use the restroom.

When I left Oregon, I promised my primary care provider I would find a new provider to continue my breast screenings while I was away. I found a provider, made an appointment, and got my mammogram. I had my old films sent for comparison and everything looked great! I had a perfect mammogram.

Once my contract was up, I found a new and bigger hospital in the area, North Shore Manhasset, and worked in the cardiology unit. This unit was still challenging but had better staffing levels. Generally, the nurse-to-patient ratio was 1:8, which was very much better than 1:13. I settled in and felt at home here with the nursing team and made some great friendships.

I moved to Long Beach, New York, while working at Manhasset. I loved the small town feel and being next to the beach. The commute to work was upwards of forty-five minutes but it didn't bother me as I found a great place to live and work. The train to Manhattan was easy to hop on and I enjoyed spending time in the city and meeting new people. I loved the New York City nightlife and thought to myself I would never leave. I finally felt alive and was having the time of my life. I met a man while I was in New York, but our relationship never advanced to the next level. I wanted more, but unfortunately it wasn't in the cards.

I decided to move on and find a new contract elsewhere. New York was getting cold, winter was settling in, and my relationship was at a dead end. I found a contract at the Mayo Clinic in Scottsdale, Arizona, and a great new apartment. I told myself I had left Oregon to find myself and should not just settle in New York—I had forty-eight other states to explore.

I made it to Phoenix in five days, traveling along Interstate 40. I thought going south was the safest bet as a snowstorm was hitting New York. I settled into my new apartment, but I wasn't able to start my new contract on time. The very first week of the new contract I had to call in sick, I apparently caught valley fever. I had no idea the water was contaminated because of the unusual rains that year. I found myself with a high fever for about three days.

Once I recovered, life started to get back to normal. I was working three twelve-hour shifts a week with four days off to find something fun to do. I traveled often when I was in Phoenix. I didn't really find a group of friends, so I spent my time in Las Vegas, back home in Oregon, New York, and I even took a trip to Florida to visit a friend. One morning in the shower I noticed a small hard lump in my left breast. It made me pause. I told myself it was nothing, but in the back of my mind I knew to keep an eye on it.

I turned thirty-one during my time in Phoenix. My coworkers thought it strange that I spent my birthday at work. That birthday was a celebration to me; I had made it to thirty-one without breast cancer. I always thought that if I made it to thirty-one, I would be fortunate enough to not walk in my mom's footsteps.

After my contract was up at the Mayo Clinic Hospital, I went back to New York and took a two-month contract in the city at the NYU Downtown Hospital. I went for a routine check-up prior to each contract, but this time I barely passed my health check. My blood work was off a little and it was puzzling to the doctor as I appeared healthy and had no complaints. He shrugged it off and passed my physical exam so I could continue to work. I was suffering with this contract as my back went out and I was having some difficulty with pain, but I made it through and decided to return back to Northshore Manhasset and return to the cardiac unit. I found a room for rent and shared a house with two other people.

A few weeks into my new permanent job and in my new place, I did another breast exam and found the same hard lump. My roommate could feel the lump, too. She worked in oncology so she made some phone calls on the spot and got me in right away to get checked out. Sure enough, at the age of thirty-one, I was diagnosed with Stage I Triple Negative breast cancer. The work-up was a whirlwind—while working at five o'clock on a Friday I learned my diagnosis from the radiology technologist. It was nice of her to let me know, but at the time I didn't have access to a doctor to help answer my questions on what my next steps should be. I was an emotional mess the entire weekend.

I decided on a lumpectomy, chemotherapy, and radiation therapy. My cousin flew in for my surgery with my father; I got to spend time with him while I recovered. The pathology confirmed I was indeed Stage I, Triple Negative Invasive Ductal Carcinoma (IDC). I had no lymph node involvement, so I felt very lucky.

I needed to prepare for chemo and hair loss. After I recovered from surgery, I took the train into Harlem and got my hair braided. I had so much fun on this little adventure and after five hours of sitting in the chair, I looked like a totally new person. I felt like this "new me" gave me new superpowers. Now I was ready to take on chemotherapy.

I was back at work after surgery. My manager collaborated with me on a schedule so I could work and do chemotherapy at the same time: I would work seven twelve-hour night shifts in a row and then walk upstairs after my night shift to receive Intravenous (IV) chemotherapy. My stepmom and niece flew in for my first appointment. I was able to spend some time with them prior to chemo, showing them around the island and enjoying the beaches and the city. I made it through my first appointment with little effects. I did have a reaction to the IV Benadryl, but otherwise I did great.

My aunt Caroline came to my second chemotherapy appointment. She flew in the day of the appointment, took a cab to the hospital, and found me sleeping in a chair when she got there. It was a really good surprise to wake up to a familiar face. She stayed with me for the week while I recovered. When I went back to work, she returned home. This was also the week I began to lose my hair and hit another emotional milestone. I was able to work through the third and fourth rounds of chemo and found support from my co-workers and roommates but after the fourth round of chemotherapy, I took a leave of absence for two months as the chemotherapy got harder and harder on my body. I felt like I had influenza body aches for the next few months and really had a hard time walking any distance. I would wake up and do my best to just get through one day at a time.

After chemo, I had radiation therapy and slowly got my strength and energy back and my life back. I spent the next three years living life as if I wasn't promised tomorrow. I decided to move back to the Pacific Northwest to be closer to family. I never really felt like I regained my health and knew deep down something was wrong, but I always had No Evidence of Disease (NED) when I went in for checkups.

For two years my health kept deteriorating. My back pain constantly flared up, and I seemed to be having heart palpitations with anxiety. Sure enough, I had a breast cancer recurrence at the age of thirty-seven. The scans and biopsies showed more than one tumor in the left breast, in the same area the original tumor was.

I decided to do a nipple-sparing mastectomy with reconstruction and chemotherapy. I went ahead with the surgery first and then chemo. The pathology resulted in triple negative in the left breast Stage I and Stage 0, the right breast had a surprise Stage 0 tumor that was ER+, and PR+. I was lucky I decided on the mastectomy, otherwise I may have had to do another treatment for the new primary tumor.

Reconstruction and chemotherapy took another year of my life, planning around appointments and feeling like I had influenza again with the main complaint being body aches and low energy. With every chemo appointment my best friend was there for me to make sure I had someone to take me, and she was the best moral support. Each time, another one of my friends or family would join in on the chemotherapy festivities. My stepsister Annette would also stay with me for about a week to make sure I was okay.

After I completed treatment the chemotherapy made me infertile and I decided to remove my ovaries as my doctors believed even though my test results for the BRACA gene variant were negative, my cancers were hereditary and ovarian cancer could be a possibility.

After recovering from removing my ovaries, I began having more and more back pain—I believe estrogen really does protect your bones. I was really struggling going to work and just doing my activities of daily living. A back fusion gave me the quality of life I had longed for. I had a horrible reaction to anesthesia and became very anemic, which lent itself to a very long recovery.

Just last year at a six-month check-up, I asked my oncologist about doing another genetic panel. Through support groups, I learned of other women who were getting their panels redone and getting answers. He agreed to do another genetic panel and, lo and behold, I received results I wasn't ready to hear. I was treating myself as if I did have a BRACA mutation, but I found out I have a TP53 mutation which is called Li-Fraumeni Syndrome.

Women with Li-Fraumeni Syndrome generally have a 100% chance of having cancer in their lifetime and oftentimes it is breast cancer. Patients with the TP53 mutation often have multiple cancers throughout their lifetimes, so knowledge is power and now I have a great plan of care that includes surveillance every year. After a skin check with my dermatologist ,a small basal cell carcinoma was removed with margins clear.

I can't stress how important it is to have a network of survivors learning from each other and supporting one another. If I didn't learn from others to really push for new genetic testing I wouldn't be on my personal path of surveillance and wellness. I personally struggled with my body image after surgeries.

Thank you to the amazing ladies I have met over the years who have helped give me the confidence to move through this precious life we only get one shot at!

Treva Vetter

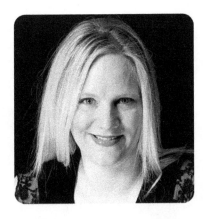

Treva Vetter has been a nurse for over 25 years and started her career as a Certified Nursing Assistant.

Treva has a Master's Degree in nursing leadership. She manages the Clinical Documentation Improvement team and the Clinical Charge Capture Analyst team st Legacy Health.

Treva takes pride in advocating for others and enjoys fundraising for non-profit organizations.

The Oregon Nurses Association honored Treva with an Economic and General Welfare award, and she has participated in Rare Disease Week on Capitol Hill.

Treva loves staying active. Her favorite travel destinations are New York and Hawaii.

"Cancer doesn't get easier, you get stronger.
Remember, life is short, buy the convertible."

Connect with Treva
Facebook: Treva Vetter

good vibes only

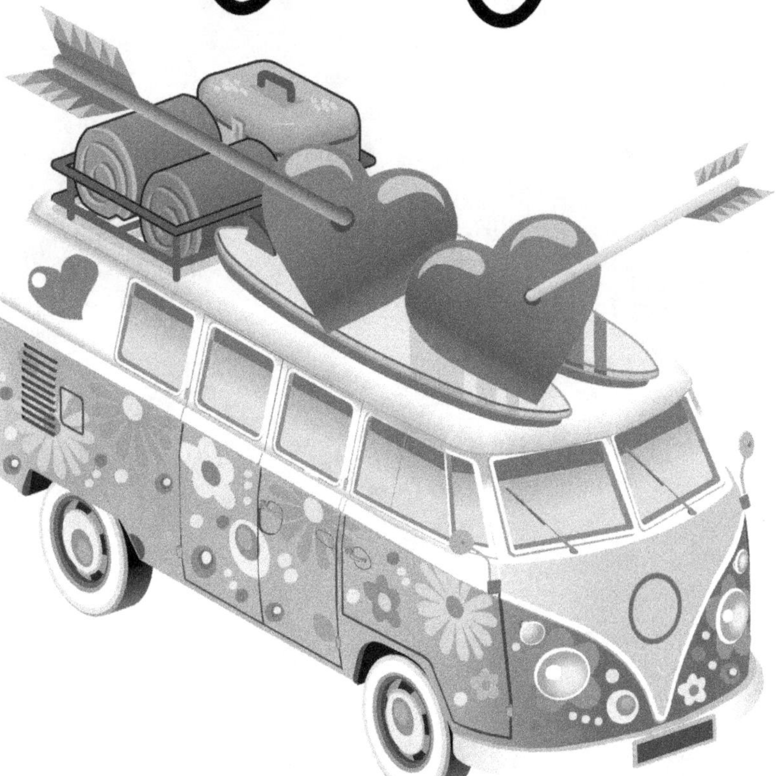

CHAPTER EIGHT
POSITIVITY HEALS
TYREEANNA HOXER

HERE I SIT in front of my computer, full of overwhelming emotions and a story that feels like both a lifetime ago and yet only just yesterday. Where to even begin I'm not sure, but here goes.

My name is Tyreeanna. I am not your average girl. I can have a mouth like a sailor at times, a quick wit, and totally lame puns. I love fishing, camping, foraging, and riding my motorcycle. I also enjoy getting dolled up, getting pampered and can't ever seem to have too many shoes, art and craft supplies, rocks, plants, or chocolate.

I grew up in a tough life, off-grid, accustomed to the nomadic lifestyle in a converted bus. From a young child, I traveled with my family, with a sense of being guided to our beautiful home base, where my parents now reside. We lived a life few people get to experience and have met so many different kinds of people along the way. I've always wanted to tell my life story to the world. It sounds like something that would be in a movie, and one day I will write a book about my travels and the experiences on our bus, known as Terrapin Bound.

My story begins in the cold winter months of November

2017; I was thirty-one years old and a mother of three beautiful children. I had been doing one of my passions, working as a preschool teacher, for about a year and had been engaged with my youngest son's dad for seven. Life was beautiful. However, the world could never prepare me for what was to come next.

One night after a long day's work, I was relaxing when I noticed my cat Jedi was following me around everywhere and would climb onto my chest as if it were his new favorite spot and purr constantly. I thought it odd at first, but then concluded he was just being super sweet and snuggly during the cold change in the weather. After a few days of my cat continuing to behave this way, lying on my chest every chance he could, I remembered watching a documentary on how animals can sense things such as the supernatural and sickness in people. That's when I decided to do a breast exam.

In the shower I noticed a lump in my left breast. I was unsure if it was something that was already there, so I thought little of it. After a few days, it started to weigh heavier on my mind, so I brought it up to my co-worker; she insisted I not delay to get in and have it looked at. Because there had been no history of cancer in my family and due to my age, the doctors thought it a cyst. It took almost two months to get me in for a mammogram.

During those two months I was in a constant state of anxiety while living in the unknown. I decided to do what I do best: I buried my fears and stress, continuing to focus on my daily life. I loved my job as a preschool teacher, it has always been one of my passions. To work with children and teach them about the world was everything to me. Spending time with babies was one of my favorite rooms to work in because I always got my snuggle fix!

Once I was able to get my mammogram, the doctors discovered this was in fact not a cyst at all. They found another lump in my other breast in the same spot and about the same size. My doctors were shocked. Those who had been working in this field their entire life had never seen anything like it. After my biopsy and blood draws, I was diagnosed with HER2+ Invasive Carcinoma in both breasts and learned I also carry the BRACA2 genetic mutation, so not only was the cancer one hundred percent estrogen fed but was also manifesting on its own at a rapid rate. Doctors told me that had I been diagnosed with this only ten years prior, it would mean a death sentence but, because of new research, immunotherapy could help with the battle. I had two chemotherapies and two immunotherapies every Friday. I had a hysterectomy, a double mastectomy, and am on hormone blockers to this day.

First of all, I just want to say I thought my tits and I were close buddies! Oh, how I was mistaken. Rather than be nice, they decided to turn against me. A dear friend/family member gave me a shirt that says, "Fondle with care," and it is by far one of my favorite shirts to this day. Every time I went in to have chemotherapy, I would wear something funny. It is so important to live life lightly and enjoy all of the little things. We are all here for a short period of time, so live it fully. I am so grateful for all of my friends and family who have rallied behind me and for everyone who supported my family and loved ones throughout those challenging times.

I was so overloaded and in shock, I had a hard time absorbing information. If it was not for both of my sisters being there for me and taking notes, I don't know what I would have done. I felt numb, almost as though I had no emotion at times. After attending counseling, I learned this was a normal response for people going through such trauma. It is a survival mode.

On March 15 after discovering I had cancer, I had to start my first chemotherapy session. Normally the surgeon would

place a port in the chest, but I got it in my arm. The port placement is done underneath the skin so when you go in for labs
and infusions, the doctor won't be required to put an IV in
every time you go in for treatments. The needle used I can best
describe as a very large thumbtack which plugs into the port.
The nurses gave me lidocaine to numb my arm before I would
come in, but I would always forget to put it on and had to just
suck it up. Therefore, the ladies who worked in labs gave me
the nickname "Tough Bitch."

I had my surgery for my port placement the day before my
first chemotherapy. I was so sore, confused, and scared and had
no idea what was going to happen. This whole world of mine
turned upside down overnight and was completely out of my
control. All I could think about was that I was not done with
my life, I needed to raise my children and was willing to do
literally anything to make it happen. I made a choice and there
was no doubt in my mind I would beat this.

As a woman, losing my hair was one of the hardest things to
go through. It is one of the ways we identify as women. I cried
many times, releasing the energy of fear, pain, and sorrow that
was constantly building up, then I would put one pant leg on at
a time and keep moving forward. I decided if my hair was to fall
out, I was going to have it go out with a bang! A dear friend of
the family who is an amazing barber gave me a pamper and
colored my hair as the rainbow. Being a preschool teacher, the
kids were thrilled when I popped into each classroom while
bouncing my hair about and shouting, "Look, I'm a pretty
pony!"

Once my hair began to fall out, my sisters again planned a
day with our amazing family/barber friend Summer for a day
of head shaving. That same day my pre-teen decided to get
lippy with me, so I looked straight into those baby blue eyes and
said, "You make me want to pull my hair out!" as I grabbed a

handful of the hair on my head and pulled out a huge clump. The look of utter shock was priceless and is forever seeded in both of our brains, no doubt!

While my head was being shaved, my sisters surprised me with the most inexpressibly beautiful and emotional moment. My sister Jeannie shaved her entire head, and my other sister Celeste shaved the back of her head and had a pink ribbon design done on it. Family and friends created a huge event for me called "Rock for the Cause." They had live bands, raffles, and prizes to help raise money for my children and me. This was done at our favorite watering hole, known as Shanahan's. The feeling of love and support I received is beyond words. It makes me tear up thinking back on it.

However, I still felt so alone even though I had so many people here for me. My relationship of seven years was going down the drain and I felt as if I was only hanging on by a thread. I found myself in a very sad place, surrounded by overwhelming darkness I had never known before. I stayed focused on the little light of my life—I am not yet finished living. I continued to push through that dark tunnel of helplessness, anger, guilt, and anxiety surrounding me that could so easily take control.

I had changed so much during that time and found myself looking at the world and others around me differently. In the grocery store, I would look at people and wonder what their story was. Anyone could take one look at me and instantly make assumptions about who I am. Yet in reality, they would have never guessed I was in pain and fighting for my life, wearing fake eyelashes, makeup to cover the redness and sores on my face, and a wig to hide from the world. I had mouth sores, bone pain, and even my fingernails were falling off due to the chemotherapy and yet somehow, I was able to find humor in almost everything. I've heard that what doesn't kill you only makes you stronger; honestly, I think it makes you funnier to boot! I was told many times someone needed to hand me a microphone.

I grew up creating art my whole life, which was how my family made a living while on the road. Everything we made we would take to events such as swap meets, Saturday markets, and farmers markets. My dad always said I had an eye and talent since I was quite young. Starting at age seven, I designed clothing and jewelry. I enjoy interacting with people and sharing what I love with the world. I continue to expand my passion to this day.

Before I got sick, I met my dear friend Dawn. She was running a farmers market in 2012 when we built a friendship, and she has always been so supportive of my work throughout these years while I continued to grow and expand my art. I taught myself how to paint while going through surgeries. It was and still is the best therapy I have ever known.

One day, I plan on providing therapy through painting and other forms of art. I want to utilize what I have been through to help other people to heal. I truly believe that inspiration and how we choose to think really does impact people when it comes to the body and healing. It's been scientifically proven that stress kills. Maybe positivity heals. I sure believe it to be true.

After being in remission for about a year, Dawn introduced me to a beautiful, strong soul. Her name is Deb, and she runs a nonprofit organization called Pink Sistas. They provide no-cost retreats for women diagnosed with breast cancer. This lady has a strength that inspires many, and she brings women together who live with the effects of cancer every day.

There is a bond that grows between the women on the retreat. Suddenly we don't feel alone, and everyone starts to share their stories. It was beautiful to be surrounded by others who truly understood what I had gone through, because they too have experienced it. She taught me how to paddle board for the very first time, and I even learned to kayak! It was great fun and filled with many laughs and wonderful memories.

Life is like a spiderweb and throughout all the good and bad times in life, it leads us to people, places, and opportunities which might never have transpired otherwise. I would not be here writing today had I not met these beautiful people on my journey called life. I am so grateful to be here today and to have this opportunity to share my story with you. Thank you for reading and I hope this will give some inspiration and light your way.

Tyreeanna Hoxer

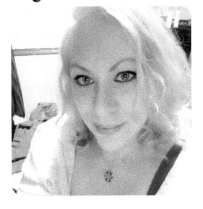

Tyreeanna Hoxer was born in Milwaukie, Oregon and her family moved to Southern California when she was one year old. It was expensive to live in California, and the family struggled to find affordable housing.

Tyreanna was just six when the family lost everything and became homeless, living in their van.

They moved to a campground in Ojai, California where they met many other homeless people. They learned about shelters, food pantries, and places where they could get clothes, new shoes, baths, and even a hot meal.

Later they settled just outside Flagstaff, Arizona, and lived completely off the grid—with no running water or electricity. The family had to haul their water and used a wood stove for heat. At age sixteen, Tyreeanna moved out, and at age twenty-one, she and her infant daughter moved to Vancouver, Washington.

She loves the outdoors and is training to forage. She is learning how to identify edible, toxic, and medicinal herbs. She designs and creates jewelry, and taught herself to paint while fighting breast cancer. She plans to help others heal through art.

Tyreeanna continues to share her incredible story and plans to write a book in the near future.

Connect with Tyreeanna
Email: Tyhoxer1986@gmail.com
Facebook: Art for the Cure: Ty's Healing Creations

I hope you feel
beautiful
today

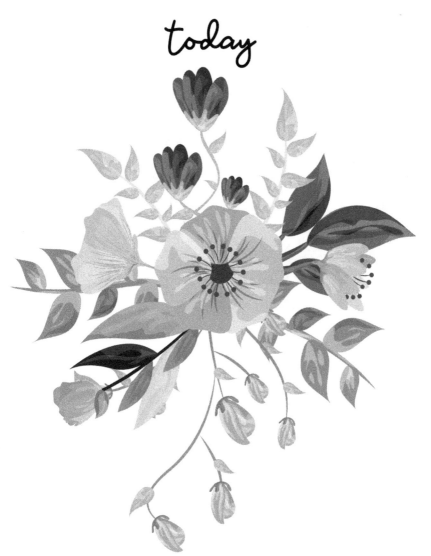

CHAPTER NINE
MY LIFE CHANGED FOREVER
KERRY FARNHAM

I NEVER THOUGHT I'd have to sit in a room like this again. Just seven years ago, my husband and I sat in a similar small conference room when we were told our eleven-year-old son's chemo treatment failed and he would not survive without a bone marrow transplant. The same, surreal, out-of-body feeling I had then came rushing back. Over the next two years, I would apply many of the lessons learned with Sam's illness to my own: reading lab reports, researching reputable sites, working with insurance, dealing with neutropenia, accepting help, and journaling.

"The results of your biopsy confirm you have Invasive Ductal Carcinoma (IDC) in both tumors." I had convinced myself it would not be cancer. After all, I was only forty-eight and there was no history of breast cancer in my family. These words knocked the wind right out of me, and I knew my life would be forever changed, again.

I was given diagrams and a report I couldn't comprehend. There would be no tears shed, not yet. Those would come later. For days and weeks after, I would lie in bed next to my husband, hoping he couldn't feel my body shake with silent sobs. But when he did, he just held me tight and let me cry.

The lady continued to explain that although this type of cancer is very common, there was a complication. Both breast tumors were HER2 positive and hormone receptor positive. She explained that HER2 meant the cancer was aggressive, and in order to have the best possible outcome, treatment would also be aggressive. She gave the analogy of a three-legged stool with each leg being a part of treatment: chemotherapy (full body and targeted), surgery, and radiation followed by hormone therapy. A whole year of my life would be spent on active cancer treatment. I had things to do, both professionally and personally. We had plans. We were going to attend my nephew's wedding in Las Vegas and see Elton John, which I had been looking forward to for almost a year. Memories of my son enduring chemotherapy consumed my thoughts. I remembered how sick he got, the excruciating pain he endured, and how utterly helpless we felt watching him suffer.

When asked where I wanted treatment, I had no idea. I had been to our small local cancer center for the first time a couple of weeks prior. I remember sitting next to a man who looked to be in his late sixties asking me what kind of cancer I had. "Oh, I don't have cancer. I'm just getting an iron infusion." It's ironic to think about that moment in time now.

I needed time to process all of this, but there was a sense of urgency in her voice. I asked her to schedule with whoever could see me first, and if I didn't feel comfortable with the doctor, I would find someone else. Three days later, on August 17, I met with Dr. Forte. I immediately knew he was the right surgeon for me.

There were people who needed to know what was happening, starting with our children. Together, we talked with our daughter, almost twelve at the time, and I told my sons. I needed to give them time to process this information too. Next, I had my husband drive me to work. I was currently on leave after having an emergency hysterectomy three weeks prior, but school was starting the next day, and when you're an elementary teacher, there are a lot of details that need to be taken care of when you are going to be gone.

Thousands of times I had walked through the front doors of the old two-story brick building where I had taught since 1991, but this time it felt different. Suddenly filled with anxiety, I was praying I would make it through the conversation I needed to have without breaking. The shock was starting to wear off and the realization of my new situation was setting in. Taking a deep breath, I walked in. The building buzzed with all of the day-before-school-starts preparations and excitement. I headed right for my principal's door and asked if we could talk in private. I took a deep breath, paused, and said those four life-changing words out loud. "I have breast cancer."

This was the third time I said those words, but the first time I cried. I am not one to cry in front of people, but there was no stopping the tears. I honestly don't remember much of our conversation, but I think he gave me a hug and told me not to worry about work. I asked him if he would read a letter from me at the staff meeting tomorrow.

I told him my diagnosis was not going to be a secret, but I wanted everyone to hear it from me. I have been known to be a control freak, and with my life in a sudden tailspin, at least I had one thing I could control.

Over the next couple of days, I shared the news with my sister, brothers, and mom. Each time I thought I was ready to say the words, "I have cancer" without crying, and each time I failed. I sought support from my friend and neighbor, another breast cancer survivor, and my dear friend Gayle, who has been battling breast cancer for decades. She was treated locally and knew all the doctors, so I leaned on her the most. Every time I had a question, she listened and gave me advice when I needed it. She kept me grounded, and every time I saw her at the cancer center, or the nurses brought me a gift Gayle had left, I felt a renewed strength. I love her dearly. I hope to use my experience and be there for others the way she has always been there for me.

The next two weeks were filled with appointments and procedures including a breast MRI, port placement, chemo school, and lymph node biopsy. Thankfully the lymph node biopsy came out clean. The chemotherapy I was going to have can cause heart issues, so I also had the first of many echocardiograms. I was thankful my days were busy. I was still healing from the hysterectomy, but I needed something on the calendar to do each day and focus on to keep from being swallowed up in my fear.

I felt very comfortable and safe with my medical team. I loved how my oncologist, Dr. Zhao, talked to us about the power of positive thinking and the important role attitude has with positive outcomes and healing. He also told us (my husband was with me and would be for almost every appointment and every chemo round) he wanted me to start an aggressive chemotherapy treatment beginning September 7. I would be given four different drugs: Taxotere, Carboplatin, Herceptin, and Perjeta. Treatment would be every three weeks for six rounds total. He gave me another stack of papers about each of these drugs.

I spent several sleepless nights reading through everything and looking up terms I didn't understand. I was careful not to read anything from "Dr. Google" and stuck to the medical sites I knew would give me the information I needed. Learning as much as I could was my way of trying to control an uncontrollable situation. Even though I was following the advice of my doctors, I wanted to be in charge of my treatment and would not follow anyone blindly.

I was also very blessed to have a nurse who recently finished treatment for triple positive breast cancer with a very similar treatment plan. I love all the nurses and staff who took care of me, but she really knew what I was feeling and fearing. She gave me insight, advice, and hope. Many tears were shed talking to Amanda, but I always felt strengthened and renewed afterward. Her survival and story helped carry me through some very dark times.

Dr. Zhao recommended having genetic testing done due to my age and lack of family history of breast cancer. This turned out to be a difficult process. Insurance refused to pay for the testing. But after three attempts and a change in the recommendation from the medical community, I finally got approval. This was very important to me, especially because I have a twin brother, a sister, and a daughter. I wanted them to have as much information as possible. It turns out I don't have any of the genetic markers that were tested for, which was a relief, but still didn't answer the question of "Why me?"

My insurance company again provided me with an amazing case manager. This was an invaluable service to us before, and I was excited to have someone help me navigate the ins and outs of cancer treatment. Charlene was an oncology nurse and a godsend. She helped me prepare for the TCHP chemo and its cumulative effects, gave terrific advice on how to help with the side effects, how to deal with insurance denials, and told me about different resources available. I took notes of every conversation, something else I had learned. This was such a valuable lesson because I would also soon learn what chemo brain is and how seriously it affects your memory. Even now, two years out, I have no recollection of conversations I had just hours before, and have trouble organizing my thoughts or finding the correct words to use when speaking. This has been one of the hardest things to cope with. I was able to deal with the horrible physical side effects because I knew it meant the chemo was working and they were only temporary. But the loss of my quick wit, ability to think on my feet, and remember conversations is something I still struggle with.

After my second round of the TCHP I lost my hair. As I walked into the appointment for my second round, Don, the CNA we all loved, commented as we walked down the hall, "How attached are you to your hair?" I knew I was going to lose it, but this was the first time we talked about it. "Well, I lost it before almost ten years ago, so I guess it will be okay." When it started falling out, my husband contacted his friend, a hair-stylist, and he cut my long curly hair short. He did this twice more over the next couple of weeks until it was all gone. The final day I did shed a few silent tears, as my adoring husband stood by my side holding my hand.

One more thing on hair: no matter how much you prepare for the loss, you still grieve. So much of our identity as women is focused on our hair, and when people see a bald woman, they see cancer. At first, I wasn't sure if I wanted to just wear hats and scarves or get a wig. I decided to do all three. For me, it was the right decision. (I like variety and choices.) Again, Charlene helped me get through this. A nice wig is expensive, and she worked very hard to get insurance to cover half the cost. I knew from my son's experience I would also lose my nose hair, which makes your nose run a lot, but I didn't think about my eyelashes and eyebrows. They go away too and looking at myself in the mirror during this time was often unbearable.

By the third round of TCHP, I wasn't sure I could go on. The bone pain, nausea, diarrhea, loss of taste, skin sores, neuropathy, and fatigue were physically and mentally debilitating. The side effects would really kick in about three days after each treatment and last for about eight days. I would then feel functional for a few days until the next round. I tried to make the most of the good days. It really does give you an appreciation for daily, mundane tasks like folding laundry, or the ability to go for a walk or meet up with a friend.

The TCHP chemo also left me neutropenic and I would often need transfusions between treatments. This took an emotional toll on us all. I am a positive person and try to always see the good in all situations. This was exhausting and frustrating. Treatment had to be postponed several times because my counts weren't high enough, and each time it was devastating. Grief and self-pity was a place I visited during these times, but I never lived there.

Cancer affects the whole family, and my heart broke for my husband. He wanted so much to take my pain away. How awful it is to watch someone you love suffer and be unable to do anything to help relieve their pain. Now he was going through it again. When I compare my experiences of going through cancer treatment myself and watching my son get sicker and weaker with each passing day, the helpless feeling of watching my son was more difficult. It was completely out of my control and I knew there was nothing I could do. At least now I had a say and was an active participant in my treatment.

I was very blessed to have a strong support system, even when treatment dragged on an extra year. My work friends gave me a hat and scarf shower, and I received weekly cards and care packages in the mail. A meal train was started, and so many prayers were said for me and my family. My colleagues donated sick leave and we were given financial support when my leave ran out and I had to start paying my insurance out of pocket. Cancer is expensive! I put my pride aside when my sister wanted to start a GoFundMe account to help with the cost of a specialty drug I would take later. As hard as it is to ask and accept help, it is necessary. All the love we received from our family, friends, community, and strangers was overwhelming at times, and I will be forever grateful. It is a very humbling experience.

I have journaled off and on since I was a teenager, so this was not a new concept for me. But my journals of the past have always been private. Many years ago, a close friend of mine told me about the Caring Bridge website. I started posting updates during Sam's illness and found the entire process very therapeutic. Now, six years later, I would start writing on Caring Bridge again. Just like before, posting proved to be healing for me, both emotionally and spiritually. I gained strength reading comments from people I loved and seeing how many "hearts" I had for each entry. It helped me feel connected to others and was a reminder I was never alone in my fight.

After the TCHP treatment was over, my husband and I met with Dr. Forte to go over the results of my latest breast MRI. The news was exactly what we had hoped for: I had a complete pathological response. We discussed surgery options and I chose a lumpectomy. On January 23, 2019, Dr. Forte removed the tissue around the tumor site along with eleven lymph nodes. Unfortunately, the margins weren't clear, and the following week I had to have surgery again to remove more breast tissue. All lymph nodes came back clear, but now I was at risk for lymphedema. I have friends who suffer with this and wanted to do everything I could to prevent it.

Charlene came to the rescue again. She told me to seek out a physical therapist who specializes in lymphedema treatment. I didn't know it was even a thing, and I would have never thought of physical therapy. She also got insurance to cover a compression sleeve. Because of this preventative treatment, I do not have any swelling on my left arm.

As soon as I was healed up enough from the surgeries, I

began thirty rounds of radiation followed by eleven rounds of targeted chemotherapy (Herceptin and Perjeta) every three weeks. It was a blessing to go through this part of treatment! My medical team was right, I had endured the worst first. I was able to go back to teaching my fourth graders on April 29, and on September 20, 2019, I finished my last chemo infusion and finally got to ring the bell.

Finishing active treatment is a strange feeling. On one hand, I was so relieved to be done and celebrated this accomplishment with my friends and family. On the other hand, it was like being adrift on a raft. I was just going where the current took me. I missed the comfort and security of going to the cancer center. I know it sounds strange, but during that time I was an active fighter. Now, I just have to wait and see, and I don't do wait-and-see very well. I needed to feel in control and actively fight any chance of recurrence. I did some more research and talked to my doctor about having an oophorectomy. Dr. Zhao, like always, supported my decision. My pathology showed a strong ER/PR component, so while this wouldn't get rid of all the hormones in my body, it would help.

When I had my hysterectomy, I didn't know I had cancer, so my ovaries were left intact. Now it was time for them to go. The surgery was successful, but I wasn't done yet. In my never-ending search for knowledge, I had become aware of a new drug used to lengthen time before recurrence for HER2+ cancers. Neratinib is an immunotherapy chemo pill I would take for one year. When I brought this up to Dr. Zhao, he wasn't too sure as the side effects can be brutal, but if it was something I wanted, he would support my decision to try. So, while I was on leave recovering from the oophorectomy, I started Neratinib on November 2, 2019.

Wow, brutal side effects was an understatement. I was bedridden for days and suffered from severe diarrhea and dehydration. My dosage was eventually reduced to a level I could tolerate, but I was still off work for two months. I was disappointed in my body for not being able to handle the full dosage because I wanted the full benefit. But I am glad to have had the opportunity to give myself every opportunity to prevent a recurrence. To counter the side effects, I had to have weekly magnesium infusions from February to November 2020. Thankfully, I could go in on Saturday mornings, so I didn't miss work. Although I'm glad I have my Saturdays free again, I do miss the "me time" those infusions gave me, and I miss seeing the nursing staff I have become so fond of.

After chemo I started on Arimidex. Because loss of bone density is a potential side effect, I had my first bone scan on December 23, 2019. I went in to establish a baseline, so I was shocked when the tech informed me I already had osteoporosis in several parts of my body. I was only forty-nine. Dr. Zhao was equally surprised and referred me to a specialist and switched me to Tamoxifen, which I have been able to tolerate well. It took almost one year to finally be seen, and I still don't have answers as to why this happened. Again, I have no family history. The specialist suggested Reclast, another infusion, to stop the progression. I agreed. I had my first infusion almost one year after the first bone scan and will have another one in a year. Just another reminder that my body will never be the same again.

PINK SISTAS

A huge source of support during all of this was our church family. Several women in our congregation are breast cancer survivors, and one dear friend suggested I join the local support group. So, in October 2018, one month after treatment started, I went to my first meeting. I knew no one there and was the only one in active treatment. These women were exactly what I needed. They were survivors and took me under their wing. I looked forward to going each month, and never missed a meeting, even when the side effects were hitting me hard.

It was at one of these meetings I first met Deb Hart. She was our speaker for the evening and told us her story of loss and cancer. I felt a connection with her immediately. She spoke about her nonprofit, Pink Sistas, and the weekend retreats for cancer survivors she hosts on her beautiful houseboat, for free! I wanted to attend; unfortunately, the retreat openings that summer were for a weekend that conflicted with a work conference in California. It would be another year before I was finally able to attend.

Because of COVID, the retreats were now just for the day, but what a glorious day it was. I met three other survivors and we ate, shared stories, did yoga, kayaked, paddle boarded (something I had always wanted to do), and went on a party boat ride. It was such a beautiful day with beautiful women and fed my soul. It was a time to just enjoy the day without any expectations, and I will forever be grateful for the experience.

Every day I think about my cancer. It's hard not to when I see the scars, pinprick tattoos from radiation, and feel the numbness at the incision sites. Cancer is a grieving process. I don't know if I will ever "get over it," but I have learned to live with it and not let it permeate every part of my life. Recurrence is still on my mind daily, but it will not stop me from living my life the best way I know how. This is hard for a control freak like me, but I am getting better at it. Each day I put it further behind me, and now my hope is to be a support for others who find themselves on this horrible cancer path.

I want to use my experience and knowledge to give hope, support, and love to other women. I will never be the person I was before cancer, but I strive to be a better version due to the lessons I learned with Sam's illness that I applied to my own. I have been on both sides: caregiver and patient. I will continue to use all my experiences to be more compassionate and empathetic to others, and especially to those who look to me for guidance and support, and that is truly a gift.

Kerry Farnham

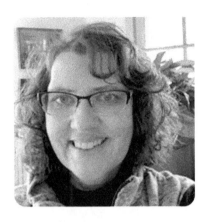

Kerry Farnham was born in Chicago, and the family moved to Montana before her first birthday.

Kerry and her twin brother, along with their younger brother and sister, grew up in a close-knit family where she learned about community service and the importance of friends.

Kerry earned her bachelor's degree from Augustana College in Sioux Falls, South Dakota, where she met Troy, her husband of 29 years. She earned a master's degree from the University of Portland and is a nationally certificated teacher. She and Troy have three children, one daughter-in-law, and one grandson.

Kerry enjoys traveling, reading, watching movies, and spending time with friends and family. She enjoys walking and hiking and loves visiting the coast. She cherishes her annual vacation with friends from high school. Kerry is an active member of her church and plays in the handbell choir with her daughter, Anna.

Kerry was diagnosed with triple-positive breast cancer at age forty-eight, with no family history. She is an advocate for breast cancer research and annual mammograms. Kerry strives to be a positive role model for others who receive a breast cancer diagnosis. She is strong in her faith and attributes her survival to her faith in God and never-ending support from her family, friends, and especially her husband, Troy.

Connect with Kerry
Facebook: Kerry Martin-Farnham

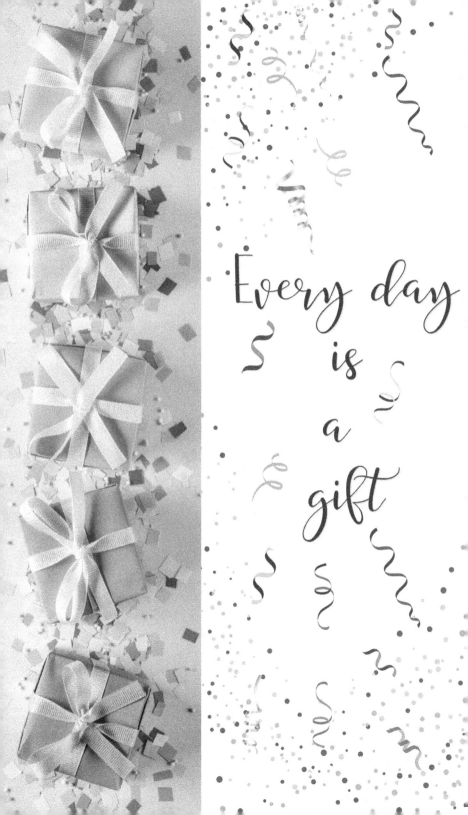

Every day
is
a
gift

CHAPTER TEN
GIFTS AND SILVER LININGS
JENNIE VINSON

My name is Jennie, and in 2014, just six days after my thirty-seventh birthday, I was diagnosed with Stage II-B Triple Positive Breast Cancer. To say this was a shock would be a complete understatement. I had an almost-three-year-old son, had just begun a new dream job at a great company, and clearly had no time for chemotherapy in my life.

Since I was so young, I had never had a mammogram. Looking back, this was most likely a mistake, as my grandmother had been diagnosed with her first breast cancer at the age of forty-one. At that time, there was no such thing as chemotherapy or radiation, so her chances of survival were slim. Her biggest fear was that she wouldn't live to be at my father's bar mitzvah, just two years away. It's the fear all mothers face when they receive a cancer diagnosis. The fear they won't be able to mother their child.

They threw the treatment book at me, starting just ten days after my diagnosis—I did six rounds of chemo over eighteen weeks, a double mastectomy, and then thirty-five radiation sessions. I decided to do reconstruction with implants, so I had to have two additional surgeries. It was definitely a marathon, not a sprint. I was very fortunate to have an amazing team of family and friends who supported me all the way through the entire process.

One thing I was able to do that I really believed help me get through all the ups and downs of treatment, was to work with a naturopath who specialized in cancer treatment. He and my oncologist collaborated on my treatment plan, so I was able to use some secondary treatments to offset some of the many side effects that I experienced. I took a ridiculous number of supplements each day, fasted in the days leading up to my chemo treatment and had Vitamin C infusions. I also had regular acupuncture and physical therapy appointments. All of these things were invaluable in supporting my quality of life, allowing me to continue to work and travel throughout most of the experience.

The other thing I believe really helped me get through my treatment was to work with a fitness trainer who focused on working exclusively with cancer patients. It felt so empowering to be lifting weights and to be moving my body. It helped me to feel alive at a time when the treatments were taking so much from me. It was amazing that I was able to increase my weight threshold throughout treatment and really great to be working out with other cancer patients.

Even with all of this support, at times during my cancer treatment fear would grip me. And to be honest, sometimes it still does even six years later. But now, instead of dwelling on the what-ifs, I've chosen to focus on the gifts and the silver linings that my cancer diagnosis and treatment haveprovided me.

From the very beginning, I knew that my cancer diagnosis had to be about something more significant. It gave me great comfort to think of my breast cancer as a teacher, a teacher that I would ask to leave my body, but a teacher, nonetheless.

I'll share some silver linings and gifts I've received in the hope that maybe you'll add these gifts to your list as you or your loved one navigates this journey.

One of my greatest gifts has been the shift of not taking any time with family, expressly my husband and son, for granted. They are my heaven on earth. I also have the best relationship with my siblings and my parents that I've ever had. There is a level of transparency and honesty I wouldn't trade for the world, and knowing the little things really aren't that big a deal. The little annoyances of life are still there, such as when the toilet seat gets left up in the middle of the night, but cancer gave me the gift of perspective. And so now I only stay mad at my husband Scott for two minutes instead of ten when sitting down on the seatless toilet. It's about progress, not perfection. Am I right?

Another gift that cancer has given is the ability to live firmly in the here and now and make the most out of every moment. It would be a bit of a cliche to say that I can do this 24/7. But I find it much simpler to do this now that I'm a cancer survivor. A few years back, my son Oscar, who is now nine years old, suggested we eat candy for breakfast. My initial instinct as a "proper" mother was, of course, to say no; but then I thought, "What would it hurt?" Soon we were sprinkling jellybeans on our oatmeal and giggling at what a treat we were sharing. His smile and his disbelief at the wonder of getting to eat candy for breakfast is something that I'll never forget. He probably won't either! And you know what? He ate more of that oatmeal than he had ever eaten before. I call that a mom win, for sure!

My breast cancer diagnosis has gifted me with the ability to lighten up about most everything and to laugh at things that would have had me crying before my diagnosis. After my first surgery, a double mastectomy, three-year-old Oscar asked me if he could see my "owies." Terror gripped me as I contemplated the fear I would inflict on his little heart when he saw the two large scars across my chest. While I was going through my treatment, my biggest worry was how this was going to impact him. But not wanting to create fear of the unknown, I slowly pulled down my tank top and showed him my chest. With wide eyes and in all earnestness, he looked at me and said, "Mama, did a ninja do that to you?"

With a huge sigh of relief and a wide grin on my face, I said, "Yes! Her name is Ninja Naik; some people call her Doctor, but we know who she really is!"

So now, my most splendid silver lining is that my son thinks that I did battle with a ninja and I won! With just a few battle scars to show for it.

One of the most cathartic silver linings about my breast cancer experience has been the certainty and comfort I have in knowing how profoundly loved I am by my family and community. Chemo and cancer changed who I am by deepening the level of intention and integrity in my life, creating discipline about what matters most, and has shone a light on my ability to persevere. My time on this grand planet is precious, and I want to make the most of every minute. I've said goodbye to laziness, goodbye to complacency, and see you later to excuses. Cancer has helped me welcome a whole new level of commitment, passion, focus, perception, consciousness, and compassion for myself, my family, and my community.

Since my diagnosis in 2014, I have been fortunate to attend a number of retreats for young breast cancer survivors. This has included learning how to surf in Maui, riding the whitewater of the Snake River, and of course the wonderful Pink Sistas retreat at the floating home on the Columbia River. Each one of these experiences has given me the ability to reflect on how far I've come and to surround myself with people who "get it" and who allow me to be right where I'm at with my feelings and my experience.

These retreats have provided me a great deal of healing, because it's not just the physical wounds that must be tended to during your cancer treatment. The emotional and spiritual wounds that the chemo can't fix have remained long after the cancer left my body. Meeting and spending time with other cancer survivors helped me to navigate this "new normal."

I'm excited to say I've met some of my best girlfriends at these retreats as a result of having had cancer. What's so nice is that as the years go by, our conversations are no longer dominated by what types of implants we have, or what our treatment schedules are. Now we are able to talk about our families and our gardens, and our hopes and dreams. We do all of this with a deep knowing of the gratitude we share for the lives we get to lead.

The gifts of cancer that have been given have been profound and are uncovered to me daily. These gifts facilitate more precious attention to the things that matter to me most and are something that, while I wish I hadn't had to have cancer to receive, I would never want to give back.

Now back to my grandmother. She did live to see my father at his bar mitzvah. She lived to see me get married and to meet my baby son. She lived until she was ninety-three. My hope is that my greatest gift will be that she and I will also share the longevity gene that she seemed to have and ultimately, the opportunity to live the long full life that she did.

Jennie Vinson

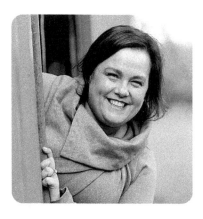

Jennie Vinson is a mom, wife, marketing consultant, and yoga instructor.

She lives with her husband Scott, 9-year-old son Oscar and her dad on a small farm in rural Oregon.

Jennie was diagnosed with Stage 2B Triple positive breast cancer in 2014 when she was 37 years old.

She enjoys cooking delicious meals, growing beautiful flowers in her garden, and looking for ways to make the world a more equitable, just place.

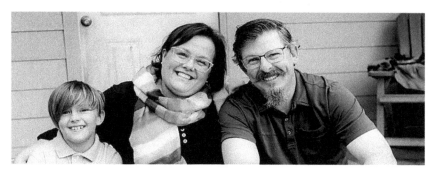

Connect with Jennie
Email: jennie@jennievinson.com
Facebook: Jennie Breslow Vinson
Instagram: @stillfiremovement or @jennieloulou
Website: www.stillfiremovement.com

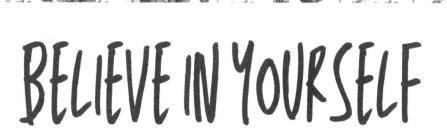

CHAPTER ELEVEN
LETTING GO OF FEAR
JANA HILL

DURING THE SUMMER OF 2015, I was working as a yoga instructor at two local gyms and as a skincare specialist at Nordstrom. Thinking back, I don't remember the exact day when I found a lump in my right breast. Finding it was a total accident; it was hard, small, and actually poked out slightly from beneath my skin. It felt like a little rock.

It's weird—I had a fear, almost an inkling, that I might get breast cancer in my life. The thought popped into my head one day several years ago and it stayed, although I didn't think about it too often. When I found the lump, I knew it was different, it was strange. I wanted to get it checked out, but I had no health insurance. I missed the window of time allotted to sign up for health insurance at my job, and now I had to wait until the end of the year.

When the time came and I was finally able to go to the doctor it was January 2016, around six months after initially finding the lump. I went in for a breast checkup, mammogram, ultrasound, and finally a biopsy. I was on my lunch break when the nurse called with the results. I was somewhat stunned to hear I had breast cancer. Stage I Invasive Ductal Carcinoma

(IDC), Estrogen Positive. I was scared and fearful. I started sobbing on the phone as my life started to flip upside down.

I was consoled by my coworkers, but I knew what I really needed was to leave work. I went home and thought about how I was going to tell my parents, friends, and family. This would be the beginning of a long road, a journey, something I had no idea how to handle. I had no idea how much my life would change over the next year. I canceled a trip to California that was coming up in just a few days. My life would become solely focused on moving forward with my battle with breast cancer.

After telling my family, I told a few close friends. One of them told me about an amazing woman named Deb Hart. She runs a nonprofit for breast cancer fighters and survivors called Pink Sistas. Deb is a breast cancer survivor herself, and she had written a book. My friend let me borrow her copy and when I opened the book to read it, I couldn't put it down. The book was well written and very interesting. It was also emotional. My friend told Deb about me, and soon Deb and I were in touch. Meeting her was wonderful and I got to learn all about Pink Sistas. They provide no-cost retreats to women diagnosed with breast cancer. I was very interested in attending but wanted to wait until after my treatment.

The first week after I was diagnosed was full of doctor appointments. Lab work, testing, MRI, surgery scheduling, meeting my oncologist—you name it, my week was packed.

After meeting with my medical team, I decided to have a double mastectomy. I would undergo chemotherapy after my surgery but no radiation. The doctor said because I was having a double mastectomy, *and* my cancer was Stage 1, I wouldn't need radiation. I was going to be given the harshest form of chemotherapy, so I was scheduled for just four treatments. Like with most things in my life, I grabbed this situation by the horns and did what I needed to do to get through it. I went nonstop and didn't look back. I followed all of my doctor's orders, changed my diet, researched heavily, and immersed myself in my fitness routine.

The biggest change I saw in myself from this was my attitude towards life and the way I lived. I let go of fear. Fear of not going after what I wanted to achieve, fear of what others thought of me, and fear of the future. Once I let go of fear and replaced it with faith, my life changed so much. If only I could have lived this way before. It took getting breast cancer for me to live my life the way I truly wanted to. I wanted to help others do the same. I also wanted to inspire others in any way that I could. I hoped I would continue living this way even after my battle was over and my life went back to normal.

After undergoing my double mastectomy, I had a breakdown. I wasn't healing well. I came home from the hospital and didn't give myself enough downtime. I was using my arms too much and moving around too soon. I ended up with a blood clot in my right breast and had to undergo emergency surgery. It was one of the hardest things I had to deal with.

I would go in for my checkups and my doctor would say, "You're just not healing well" or he would say, "It's taking longer than usual for you to heal." It was frustrating because I was doing everything I was supposed to do. I was taking really good care of myself. It felt like an eternity as I laid in bed, trying to heal. A friend of mine told me to be patient and love your body, it's working hard for you right now. Those words helped me a lot.

When I was feeling better, I started tissue expansion every two weeks to prepare my body for breast implants. Once I was healed enough, I started working out again, gently. I eased into it and I continued teaching my yoga classes.

Yoga and fitness were my saving grace. Instead of staying home and being depressed, I got myself to the gym and worked out when I could. I was on a pretty regular schedule and feeling really good. I was in even better shape than I was before I was diagnosed with breast cancer. I was starting to inspire people around me which felt amazing. That's when I started thinking about working as a personal trainer. It's something I had thought about for years but never pursued. I kept it in the forefront of my mind.

I began my chemotherapy treatments soon after I recovered from the mastectomy surgery. They were scheduled every three weeks. It was tough because I had to take medication, give myself shots, and continue with the tissue expansion. I was also dealing with the side effects of the chemo. I prevailed and stayed strong with my workouts and teaching yoga.

There were many days when I felt so horrible, I didn't think I could bear teaching my yoga class, going to the gym, or even getting out of bed. Most of the time I *forced* myself to go. It wasn't easy, but by the time I was done, I felt so much better. Wow, I had really proven to myself that I was stronger both mentally and physically than I thought. If I could do this, so could others who are going through the same thing.

I eventually lost all my hair, started wearing scarves, and got a really cute wig. During this time, I was invited to be a part of the Pink Sistas annual calendar that would be published the following year. The photoshoot was a lot of fun, the photographer took pictures of me on a paddle board. It was my first time on one, and I was so nervous! We also went out on a beautiful yacht for some really fun pictures.

As I was nearing the end of my chemo treatments, I began to seriously consider working as a personal trainer. I started my studies and trained at a fitness facility in Happy Valley, Oregon. I loved it there and it felt like family. The environment was awesome, and I felt like I was in my element. By the end of Summer 2016, I was working as a personal trainer and as a yoga instructor. I was happy. My story not only inspired others but motivated them as well.

It was around this same time I finished my chemotherapy and tissue expansions. I was preparing for my breast implant surgery that was scheduled for the end of September. I got myself really strong before surgery and allowed myself plenty of time for healing. I had built up a clientele and started growing my social media platforms. It's always hard taking breaks from life when you have to have surgery, but I allowed myself that time to relax and not be too hard on myself. I knew I could pick back up where I left off, and if I let go of that fear and held onto my faith, everything would be okay.

Once I was healed, I felt like it was the perfect time to go on a Pink Sistas Retreat. I went on a weekend retreat in Pine Hollow, Oregon. It was such a great time. Meeting other ladies and connecting with women who had been through the same or similar situations as myself. Everyone was wonderful and Deb was a great hostess. The food was incredible. We did a lot of different activities: jewelry making, hiking, and fellowship. I even led the ladies in a yoga class! Pine Hollow was beautiful and relaxing. I felt a lot of gratitude that weekend.

After I got home from the retreat, I had to prepare for another surgery. I needed another breast augmentation as the first one left my breasts very uneven and different sizes. This surgery would include fat grafting to make my breasts more even. I also elected to have nipple reconstruction. I've been a little bit of a perfectionist my whole life, so it was hard not having beautiful breasts. But after going through this experience, I humbled myself and accepted that my breasts would never be perfect.

The last and hopefully final surgery I had was a full hysterectomy. That was a really hard surgery for me. It took a while to feel "normal" again.

About a year after my hysterectomy, I participated in a fashion show fundraiser for Pink Sistas. My daughter and I were models in the fashion show, and my son came along, too. We had a yummy lunch after the show, and all for a great cause!

Pink Sistas biggest fundraiser of the year is their annual Pink in the Gorge auction. They have a silent auction, live auction, live band, food, and fun! I was so excited I could attend the auction and support Pink Sistas.

Last summer, I went to a day retreat with Pink Sistas on their houseboat on the Columbia River. We had a full day. We went boating on the river, and then paddle boarding and kayaking out by the boat houses where the river currents were quieter. I was so proud of myself because I was able to stand up on the paddle board! It was so much fun being on the water and meeting new friends. I'll always be grateful for my amazing experiences with Pink Sistas.

There always seems to be something positive you can take from negative situations. For me, it was getting involved with Pink Sistas and making new friends as well as growing friendships I already had.

Being diagnosed and dealing with breast cancer has changed my life for the best. Going forward, I just want to live my life with love and be the healthiest, happiest version of myself!

Jana Hill

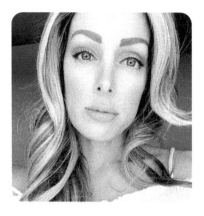

Jana Hill is a mother, yoga instructor, and aesthetician.

Her children mean everything to her and she loves living life to its fullest.

Jana's hobbies include reading, working out, and photography. Her favorite way to enjoy her time is with her family.

Jana received her diagnosis of Stage 1 breast cancer at age thirty-seven. Jana was working as a personal trainer and yoga instructor at the time. Keeping active in her health and fitness was her saving grace. It helped her to deal with the emotional and physical side effects of chemotherapy and fighting cancer.

Jana is nearing her five-year mark of being cancer-free.

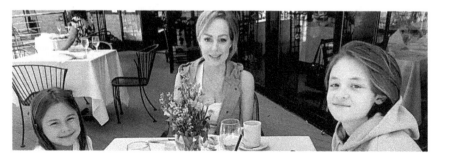

Connect with Jana
Email: Janaleehill@gmail.com
Instagram: @janaleefitness
Instagram: @beautybyjanalee

Once you choose hope, anything is possible

CHAPTER TWELVE
THERE IS HOPE
KIMMI ALEXANDER

Sitting here writing about my life is no easy task.

I went from fit, active, full of energy, and healthy to being diagnosed with breast cancer in the summer of 2017, after finding a lump while in the shower.

After two months of the doctor sending the wrong orders to the Kearney Breast Center, we were finally able to get in for a mammogram. At the appointment, the doctor explained they needed a biopsy for confirmation of what appeared to be cancer. I left the appointment feeling confident that again this was nothing to worry about.

I was wrong.

Stage II Invasive Ductal Carcinoma (IDC), PR+ ER- and HER2- was the diagnosis and I was scheduled for a biopsy the following week. Again I felt no reason to take anyone with me; I had an "I can do this myself" attitude. I was greeted by the doctor, the ultrasound technician, and two other lovely young ladies who were so wonderful to have there. They held my hand and talked me through everything. As the appointment went on, their findings became evident.

This was on a Wednesday, and it had to be forwarded to

pathology and then to my doctor. It was a difficult couple of days, just wondering what was happening. On Friday at 4:54 p.m., my doctor called to say, "Kimmi, your results show you have breast cancer." It felt like the longest phone call, when in reality it was probably just a couple of minutes.

She was sorry to have to give me the news but would get me set up with a cancer center. She wished me luck and said she would follow up and be there for me.

When I got off the phone, it felt so unreal—all the emotion and questions: what if, where do I go, what's going to happen, how am I paying for this, what about my work, and more. The flood of uncertainty came rushing in. I just didn't know anything.

At that point we decided to tell the family. I'm very close to my parents, and being the only daughter, I knew telling them would probably be the most difficult. I didn't want to cause them any stress. My mom was a two-time breast cancer survivor; she dug in her heels and went through it like it was a breeze. She never talked about it. All she could tell me was, "I'm so sorry, and I wish I could take your place." She and my father were devastated. I told her, "Mom, you did it, and I can do this. It's okay! I'm going to be okay."

Next, we told my three grown kids. My oldest daughter Nikki and two oldest grandkids were immediately en route from Idaho to be here, dogs in tow. My middle daughter and son were pretty numb, and not wanting to talk about it. They still don't talk much about it.

A few days later the cancer center called to set me up with my new doctor. Wow, so much to absorb! They quickly made an appointment for markers to be put in and for more tests. So much to do. So many questions, so much anticipation and worry.

My appointment came with my surgeon, what a breath of

fresh air! She meticulously went over everything step-by-step with a positive attitude. *We've got this!*

We saw that the same tumor had been on the other, prior films. She felt my cancer was slow growing and had been there for a while. She remained confident, so here we go.

I met my new team. I was loaded down with information, a book of appointments, testing, and scans. An appointment for another doctor! What's that for? He was another member of my team, a plastic surgeon—what the heck? But what a pleasure it was to meet him and his staff. They went over everything in great detail and were very caring.

Even so, I left both appointments feeling overwhelmed. I felt so lost with worry. I was scheduled for a double mastectomy in August. I got through it, and wow, what a process! My mom, dad, and my boyfriend Ed were all there for my surgery. When I woke up, I felt like a football player with huge shoulder pads, and I felt as if a Mack truck had hit me! I had machines hooked up to me and drains sticking out of me.

Now the healing begins.

I was sent home the next day and did surprisingly well. The house was well prepared for my recovery. I didn't think about what I wouldn't be able to do—I just concentrated on making sure the house was prepared. And the house was—but I wasn't.

It was difficult, but I managed to move along in my recovery. The sight of myself after mastectomy wasn't something I was ready for. It wasn't pretty at all; I was not at all prepared in my head for that part. I had no nipples, and my chest looked like something out of a bad dream.

The day the bandages came off, I thought I would never feel whole again. Ed was in charge of my dressings and drains; he had to record the fluid output from the drains. He was awesome, being he's not very empathetic and has a very weak stomach. He is a sport fisherman night and day, so I wasn't sure how he would survive it—but he was a true warrior beside me, making sure I was safe and caring for my every need.

Next came more appointments, follow-ups, tests, and more surgeries. Expanders were placed at the same time as the mastectomy to prepare for reconstruction surgery. After a period of time, they started to fill the expanders, and it was another experience to say the least! They prepared my skin, and then I was scheduled for another surgery in December.

To our family's dismay, my beautiful mother, best friend, our everything—passed away in her sleep on Friday, December 9, from a heart attack. I thought, "This can't happen, it's not real." There was no warning. We had just left their home, one mile from our house. I was a mess; I just couldn't believe it. The guilt hit me—was it from the worry she carried for me that caused this? It's been a whirlwind; I still can't believe she is gone. I am feeling defeated going through all this without her, not wanting to go through with any of this anymore.

I had my second surgery shortly after she passed. It was difficult without her there, but I pushed through. My Oncotype score came back at twenty-seven, and for now I've decided not to go through chemo. I'm not ready to go through this without my mom here with me.

I continued with the rebuild. Implants for breast cancer patients are *not* the same as having a boob job. First, there is the removal of our tumor (or tumors) and surrounding breast tissue. From there, we are rebuilt from the inside out. Fine-tuning means more surgeries; fat grafting, revision, and for some, tattoos. Believe me, these doctors are perfectionists!

I went from feeling botched and scarred from one end to another, to feeling confident again. Then came the finishing touches. I was blessed meeting Casey White, a tattoo artist who flew in from California to gift me my 3D "tit tats."

This was another experience that wasn't quite what I was expecting. I had no idea there was an option to have your nipples tattooed. Again, top-notch treatment, and Casey has just a huge heart for women going through this.

I think dealing with the side effects has been the worst part about having breast cancer. My teeth have cracked, and my bones are disintegrating. The brain fog comes and goes. I have phantom pains and neuropathy.

In August 2020, I took a bad fall due to low blood pressure and because my potassium levels had dropped. I felt a snap, and then I could hear static (like on television) in my head. Knowing I smacked my face on the counter on the way down was a big "dang it" moment. I was hurting but washed my face, brushed my teeth, and went to bed.

I woke up feeling very sore. Ed took one look at me and said, "Come on, we have to get to the hospital!" I was dumbfounded. I had hemorrhaged during the night, my eye was swollen shut, and the right side of my face was unrecognizable. He took me to our local hospital, and they quickly transferred me to the OHSU Trauma Center. What the heck? I was greeted by a team of doctors and nurses in full gear who were ready for me.

Long story short, when I hit my face, I had ended up with several fractures. So, off to another surgery I went. This time, though, it was for my face. They had to insert two titanium plates, and they weren't able to save the eyesight in my right eye. I am now permanently blind in my right eye, but they were able to save the eyeball itself. So, I have that to be thankful for. The optic nerve can't be fixed. I don't understand why they can do everything else, but not fix the optic nerve. It's frustrating . . . it feels like I'm in a never-ending story, and it's been hard to wrap my head around it.

But I'm alive, and thankful to all who have helped me

through these critical times. It hasn't been easy to absorb everything. But I know without this team on my side, I would have fallen apart. I have one hundred percent faith in my cancer team. They were my saving grace. People ask me how I'm getting through everything, and I tell them the cancer is for my doctors to worry about. I just need to be thankful and not overthink any of it. They have taken my fear away.

This is just a tiny bit of what we go through, there's so much more to it. The discomfort caused by the medications, infusions, and treatments does not go away. We don't know what to expect next. Every day is a new day. As we reflect on our journey, we must never lose faith in ourselves and the willpower we have to get through and fight on!

I am thankful for Deb Hart and her nonprofit organization, Pink Sistas. They do so much to help women diagnosed with breast cancer to help us overcome what we may be going through or are still facing. I have not yet been able to join in on her many adventures or retreats she offers, but after the COVID restrictions are lifted, I will be joining in. Thank you, Deb, for bringing us together.

For anyone about to go through this journey, YOUR FIGHT IS OUR FIGHT! You are not alone. Talk about it and reach out, we are all in this together. As bad as it is, there is hope.

Kimmi Alexander

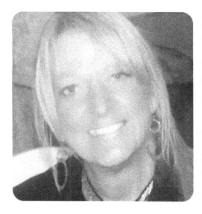 Kimmi Alexander is a healthcare worker and spends her time giving compassion to heal the heart and ease the pain of those in need at end of their life's journey.

Losing her mother, and just recently, her son-in-law has been the hardest moments in her life so far.

Kimmi raised her three children in Alaska. Later, she moved to Washington to be near her mother and father. With luck on their side, she and her boyfriend Ed found a dream home within a mile of her parents. Her three children and nine grandchildren live nearby and are part of her everyday life.

Kimmi's family comes first and they are her number one priority. She and Ed provide a loving atmosphere for all who come through their door. They welcome friends and family with open arms. There is never a dull moment!

She enjoys spending time fishing, playing poolside, traveling, entertaining, and making people laugh. Nothing can stop her.

"The sky is the limit to anything you set your mind to."

Connect with Kimmi
Email: Kimmialexander@gmail.com
Facebook: Kimmi Alexander

Life is a journey, not a destination

CHAPTER THIRTEEN
PAUSE, REFLECT, AND PIVOT
DEB HART, FOUNDER OF PINK SISTAS

WHEN I FOUNDED PINK SISTAS, my vision was to provide a weekend getaway where women who have breast cancer could be pampered and wouldn't have to think about their diagnosis for a few days. The idea evolved into offering the opportunity to relax, unwind, experience new things, and to connect with others who are there or who have been there, in a unique way that leaves a lifetime of memories.

I'm so proud to say Pink Sistas is one hundred percent run by volunteers, we do not have any paid staff, including myself. For the first time in ten years, our current board of directors are all breast cancer survivors. Each woman brings her own unique expertise and is passionate about Pink Sistas and supporting women diagnosed with breast cancer.

We served over ninety women in 2019 and had great plans for 2020—until COVID hit. We were preparing for our biggest fundraisers of the year and had to make some tough decisions. Our two biggest events, the live auction and golf tournament, would not be held in 2020.

Our annual auction, *Pink in the Gorge*, has traditionally been an in-person event. With a silent auction, dinner, live auction, and live music, it has always been a sparkling, fun-filled evening! But now because of COVID, we couldn't hold a live event because everything was shutting down. And most importantly, because cancer compromises your immune system, there was absolutely no way I could hold an event and take the chance even one person would become sick.

I had to pause and take a close look at how we were operating versus how we needed to pivot in order to keep going. We needed to figure out a different way. What was Pink Sistas going to look like without our regular in-person fundraising events?

The first thing we did was research how to replace our live auction with a virtual auction. It was a big job, but we made it work. We found a company to work with and our volunteers stepped up to make everything run smoothly. We found out through trial and error what worked and what wasn't so great.

We launched a book, *Waves of Pink: Stories of Sisterhood*. It became one of our biggest fundraisers to date. And it was so successful, we decided to do another book—and you're reading it now. Sharing our stories is important. Knowing there is someone who has gone through the same thing can be so comforting. And it is therapeutic; this is the first time some of these women have told their story.

I had to pause again and figure out how we could move forward with our retreats. I met with one of my mentors, Jan Westin. He is a successful businessman and a strong supporter of Pink Sistas. His company, Westin Kia, is one of our original corporate sponsors.

We had a conversation around how I could shift the way Pink Sistas served women. Jan said to me, "You still have the boat, you can still kayak and paddle board. What if you just have guests come for the day instead of the weekend." There was our pivot.

To be really honest, once we started doing the day retreats, I heard from several different people that they had always wanted to go to the weekend retreats, but after being gone from family for treatments and doctor appointments, they felt guilty leaving for a weekend away from home. Plus, anyone with children had to worry about childcare for the weekend getaway. It was easier for the women we serve to get away for just one day.

So, we revamped our retreats. We are excited to have fifteen retreats scheduled in 2021. There are twelve retreats for survivors, and three couples retreats. We paddle boarded, kayak, have an amazing lunch, and a boat ride on the beautiful Columbia River. Relax, refresh, connect.

Taking time to *pause* and *reflect*, and then if needed, *pivot*. These three words helped to keep Pink Sistas operational during the pandemic. We will carry on with new ideas and continue our mission to support women who have been diagnosed with breast cancer.

For more information on how you can support Pink Sistas, please visit www.pinksistas.org.

Deb Hart

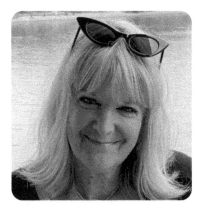

Deb Hart is the founder of Pink Sistas, Inc.

Deb is an inspirational speaker, mother, mentor, friend, breast cancer survivor, and breast cancer survivor confidant.

Pink Sistas is a 501(c)3 non-profit corporation dedicated to raising funds for no cost retreats for women who have been diagnosed with breast cancer.

Pink Sistas retreats focus on healing after diagnosis of breast cancer through many activities: networking with others, yoga, art, kayaking and paddle boarding, social outings, and much needed rest and relaxation.

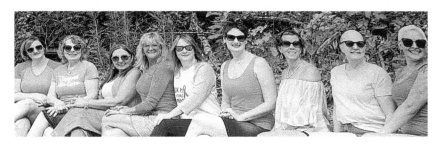

Connect with Deb
Email: inspirationaldebhart@msn.com
Facebook: Pink Sistas, Inc
Website: https://pinksistas.org
Website: https://www.inspirationaldebhart.com

ACKNOWLEDGMENTS

Pink Sistas would like to extend our utmost gratitude to the people and businesses who support our mission.

In your lifetime, you will meet people who will stand with you. If you're fortunate, you will intersect with people who will not only stand with you, they will champion your cause and cheer for you each time you triumph.

Please support the businesses on the following pages, they are advocates for women with breast cancer, and they have partnered with us to help bring this book to you. They are our champions and if you listen very carefully, you might just hear them cheering.

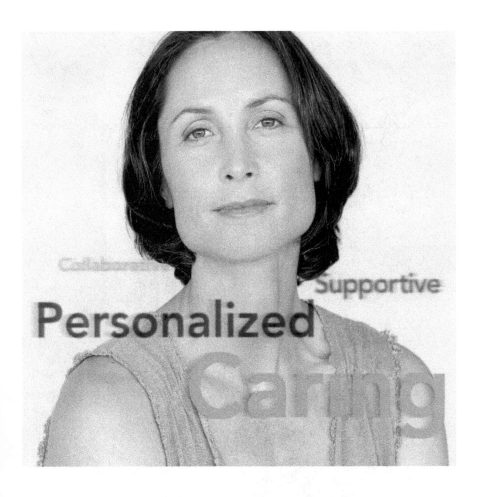

Collaborative

Supportive

Personalized

Caring

Cancer care built around you

Compass Breast Specialists is a multidisciplinary team of surgical, medical and radiation oncologists, nurse navigators and supportive care experts. From the beginning of treatment to life beyond cancer, you'll find a culture of listening, collaboration and respect.

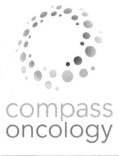

compass
oncology

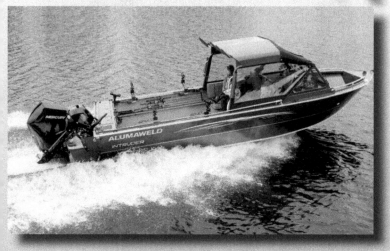
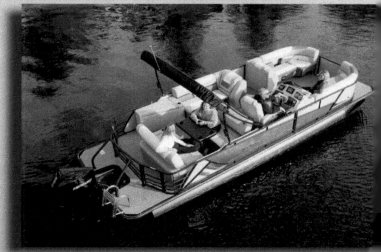

I am a breast cancer _Thriver!_

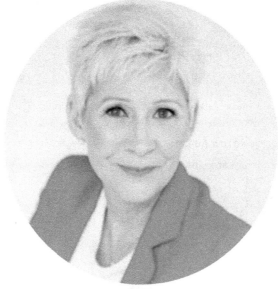

Lori Godfrey

"Let's make something positive happen today."

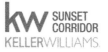

REAL ESTATE GROUP

kw SUNSET CORRIDOR
KELLERWILLIAMS.

Principal Broker-Owner
Five Star Agent, Awarded 2011 - 2021

lorigodfrey@kw.com
www.thegodfreyrealestategroup.com

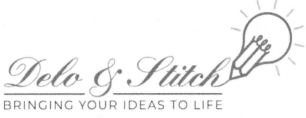
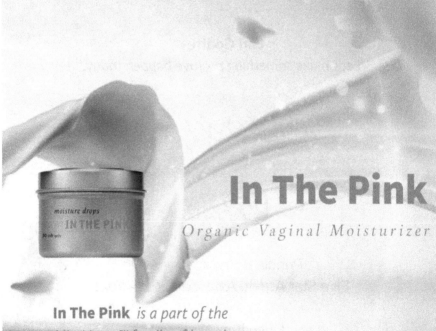

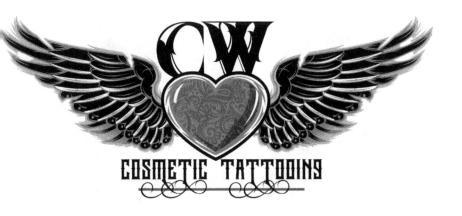

COSMETIC TATTOOING

"It's More Than Just a Tattoo"

One goal in mind...
YOU

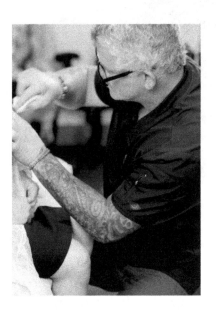

Cosmetic Tattooing

Inclusive

Areola Tattooing

Permanent Makeup

Scalp Micropigmentation

CW Cosmetic Tattooing
Paramedical Permanent Cosmetics
Located in Southern California

(714) 925-0601
www.cwcosmetictattooing.com

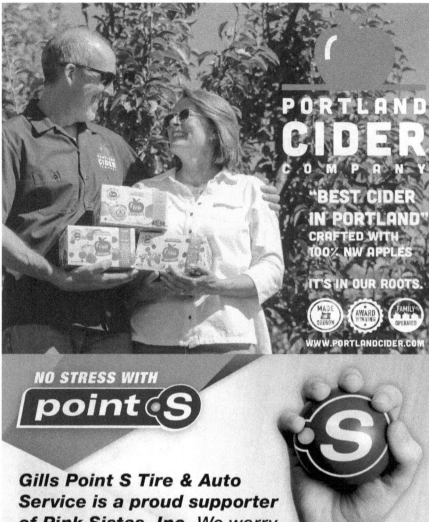
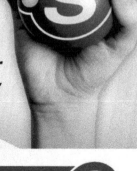

CORPORATE SPONSOR

WESTON
BUICK KIA GMC

We would like to sincerely thank Weston Kia, our very first corporate sponsor. Weston Kia and Pink Sistas have been in partnership for ten years. We are incredibly grateful for their support and generosity. Jan Weston has become a great friend and wise mentor.

Jan Weston and the Weston Kia family donated our party boat, the TICKLED PINK. Weston Kia sponsors our annual fundraising event, Pink in the Gorge as well as the Pink Sistas calendar.

Thank you, Jan Weston and Weston Kia!

CORPORATE SPONSOR

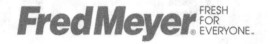

Fred Meyer has been a valued corporate sponsor of Pink Sistas for nine years. They are a presenting sponsor for our Pink in the Gorge annual fundraiser, and they provide all of our printing needs, including the Pink Sistas calendars. They also generously donate swag bags for all of our retreat guests.

Each year, Fred Meyer sponsors a Pink Sistas weekend retreat for employees of Fred Meyer who have been diagnosed with breast cancer.

Thank you, Fred Meyer!

CORPORATE SPONSOR

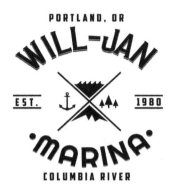

Will-Jan Moorage is a floating home marina on the Columbia River in Portland, OR.

Brian and Randi Norton are third-generation owners and are happy to support Pink Sistas by hosting the Pink Sistas party boat for their day retreats.

Randi has been a dedicated Oncology nurse for nearly ten years. Supporting cancer survivors is an important part of thier daily lives, and offering support through the Marina is an extra blessing.

We look forward to Wil-Jan Marina hosting Pink Sistas retreats starting in 2021!

Thank you for your generosity, Wil-Jan Marina!

HOW YOU CAN HELP

Pink Sistas is dedicated to honor, support, and help women affected by a diagnosis of breast cancer. We would not be able to serve our community of women without your generous donations and continued support.

Your donations allow us to continue our mission by providing important resources, new venues for our retreats, and increase breast cancer awareness in our community.

To donate, sponsor, or volunteer, please visit:
https://www.pinksistas.org/howyoucanhelp

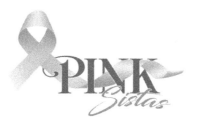

GLOSSARY

ABRAXANE

Abraxane typically is used to treat advanced-stage breast cancer and usually is given in combination with other chemo-therapy medicines or after other chemotherapy medicines given after surgery have stopped working

ALLODERM

Alloderm is a biologic mesh-like material derived from animals or donated (cadaveric) human skin. It is used in many different types of reconstructive surgery including breast reconstruction.

AROMATASE INHIBITOR

Aromatase inhibitors stop the production of estrogen in post-menopausal women. Aromatase inhibitors work by blocking the enzyme aromatase, which turns the hormone androgen into small amounts of estrogen in the body. This means that less estrogen is available to stimulate the growth of hormone-receptor-positive breast cancer cells.

ATYPICAL EPITHELIAL HYPERPLASIA

Atypical hyperplasia is a precancerous condition that affects cells in the breast. Atypical hyperplasia describes an accumulation of abnormal cells in the milk ducts and lobules of the breast. Atypical hyperplasia isn't cancer, but it increases the risk of breast cancer.

AXILLARY NODE DISSECTION

An axillary lymph node dissection (ALND) is surgery to remove lymph nodes from the armpit (underarm or axilla). The lymph nodes in the armpit are called axillary lymph nodes. An ALND is also called axillary dissection, axillary node dissection or axillary lymphadenectomy.

BIOPSY

A biopsy is a procedure to remove a piece of tissue or a sample of cells from your body so that it can be analyzed in a laboratory.

BRCA1 AND BRCA2 (BRCA1/2) GENE MUTATIONS

Genes that help limit cell growth. A mutation (change) in one of these genes increases a person's risk of breast, ovarian, and certain other cancers. Everyone has BRCA1 and BRCA2 genes.

CARCINOMA

Cancer that begins in the skin or in tissues that line or cover internal organs.

CHEMO BRAIN

A term commonly used to describe thinking and memory problems that a patient with cancer may have before, during, or after cancer treatment. Signs and symptoms of chemo brain include disorganized behavior or thinking, confusion, memory loss, and trouble concentrating, paying attention, learning, and making decisions.

Chemo brain may be caused by the cancer itself (such as brain tumors) or by cancer treatment, such as chemotherapy and other anticancer drugs, radiation therapy, hormone therapy, and surgery. It may also be caused by conditions related to cancer treatment, such as anemia, fatigue, infection, pain, hormone changes, sleep problems, nutrition problems, stress, anxiety, and depression. Chemo brain may last for a short time or for many years.

CYTOXAN

Cytoxan (cyclophosphamide) is a cancer (chemotherapy) medication used to treat several types of cancer.

DIEP FLAP RECONSTRUCTION

A type of breast reconstruction procedure. During DIEP flap reconstruction surgery, a surgeon will take healthy tissue, skin, and fat from the person's lower abdomen to use in breast reconstruction.

DUCTAL CARCINOMA IN SITU

If cancers arise in the ducts of the breast (the tubes that carry milk to the nipple when a woman is breastfeeding) and do not grow outside of the ducts, the tumor is called ductal carcinoma in situ (DCIS). DCIS cancers do not spread beyond the breast tissue. However, DCIS may develop over time into invasive cancers if not treated.

EARLY BREAST CANCER

Cancer that is contained in the breast or has only spread to lymph nodes in the underarm area. This term is often used to describe Stage 1 and Stage 2 breast cancer.

ENCAPSULATED

Confined to a specific, localized area and surrounded by a thin layer of tissue.

EXCISIONAL BIOPSY

A surgical procedure in which an entire lump or suspicious area is removed for diagnosis. The tissue is then examined under a microscope.

HER2-POSITIVE (HER2+) BREAST CANCER

In about 20% of breast cancers, the cells make too much of a protein known as HER2 (Human Epidermal Growth Factor Receptor 2, HER2/neu, erbB2). These cancers tend to be aggressive and fast-growing.

HER2-negative (HER–) breast cancers have little or no

HER2 protein. HER2-positive (HER+) breast cancers have a lot of HER2 protein. HER2+ tumors can be treated with HER2-targeted therapies, such as trastuzumab (Herceptin).

HER2 POSITIVE OR NEGATIVE

About 10% to 20% of breast cancers depend on the gene called *human epidermal growth factor receptor 2 (HER2)* to grow. These cancers are called "HER2 positive" and have too many HER2 receptors and/or extra copies of the *HER2* gene. The *HER2* gene makes a protein that is found on the cancer cell and is important for tumor cell growth. A breast cancer that does not have excessive numbers of HER2 receptors or copies of the *HER2* gene is called "HER2 negative."

HERCEPTIN

A drug used alone or with other drugs to treat certain types of breast cancer, stomach cancer, and gastroesophageal junction cancer that are HER2 positive. It is also being studied in the treatment of other types of cancer. Herceptin binds to a protein called HER2, which is found on some cancer cells. This may help the immune system kill cancer cells. Herceptin is a type of monoclonal antibody and a type of HER2 receptor antagonist.

HORMONE RECEPTOR POSITIVE OR NEGATIVE

Breast cancers expressing estrogen receptors (ER) and proges-terone receptors (PR) are called "hormone receptor positive." These cancers may depend on the hormone's estrogen and/or progesterone to grow. A breast cancer that does not have estrogen and progesterone receptors is called "hormone receptor negative".

INFLAMMATORY BREAST CANCER (IBC)

A rare, aggressive form of invasive breast cancer whose main symptoms are swelling (inflammation) and redness of the breast. The skin on the breast may look dimpled, like the skin of an orange, and may be warm to the touch.

INVASIVE DUCTAL CARCINOMA (IDC)

IDC, also known as infiltrating ductal carcinoma, is cancer that began growing in a milk duct and has invaded the fibrous or fatty tissue of the breast outside of the duct. IDC is the most common form of breast cancer, representing eighty percent of all breast cancer diagnoses.

LI-FRAUMENI SYNDROME (LFS)

Li-Fraumeni syndrome (LFS) is an inherited familial predisposition to a wide range of certain, often rare, cancers. This is due to a change (mutation) in a tumor suppressor gene known as TP53. The resulting p53 protein produced by the gene is damaged (or otherwise rendered malfunctioning), and is unable to help prevent malignant tumors from developing.

Individuals with LFS have an approximately 50% of developing cancer by age 40, and up to a 90% percent chance by age 60, while females have nearly a 100% risk of developing cancer in their lifetime due to their markedly increased risk of breast cancer. Many individuals with LFS develop two or more primary cancers over their lifetimes.

LUMPECTOMY (BREAST CONSERVING SURGERY)

Breast surgery that removes only the tumor and a small rim of normal tissue around it, leaving most of the breast skin and tissue in place.

MARGINS

The rim of normal tissue surrounding a tumor that's removed during breast surgery.

A margin is clean (also known as uninvolved, negative or clear) if there's only normal tissue (and no cancer cells) at the edges. Clean margins show the entire tumor was removed.

With involved (positive) margins, normal tissue doesn't completely surround the tumor. This means the entire tumor was not removed and more surgery may be needed to get clean margins.

MASTECTOMY

Surgical removal of the breast. The exact procedure depends on the diagnosis.

METASTASES

If any cancer is detectable outside of the breast, these deposits are called metastases.

METASTATIC BREAST CANCER

Breast cancer that has spread beyond the breast to other organs in the body (most often the bones, lungs, liver or brain).

Metastatic breast cancer is not a specific type of breast cancer, but rather the most advanced stage (Stage 4) of breast cancer.

N.E.D.

No evidence of disease (NED) is often used with cancer when there is no physical evidence of the disease on examination or imaging tests after treatment. No evidence of disease means the same thing as complete remission or complete response. It does not, however, mean that a cancer is cured.

NEULASTA

A drug that is used to prevent infection in adults and children with neutropenia (a lower-than-normal number of white blood cells) caused by anticancer drugs that may stop or slow the growth of blood-forming cells in the bone marrow. Neulasta helps the bone marrow make more white blood cells.

NEUTROPENIA

Neutropenia is when a person has a low level of neutrophils. Neutrophils are a type of white blood cell. All white blood cells help the body fight infection. Neutrophils fight infection by destroying harmful bacteria and fungi (yeast) that invade the body.

ONOCTYPE SCORE

The Oncotype DX test is a genomic test that analyzes the activity of a group of twenty-one genes from a breast cancer tissue sample that can affect how a cancer is likely to behave and respond to treatment.

OOPHORECTOMY

Surgery to remove one or both ovaries.

PERI MENOPAUSE

Peri menopause, or menopause transition, begins several years before menopause. It's the time when the ovaries gradually begin to make less estrogen. It usually starts in women's 40s, but can start in their 30s or even earlier.

PERJETA

A drug used with other drugs to treat HER2 positive breast cancer. It is used in patients whose cancer has spread to other parts of the body and has not already been treated with other anticancer drugs. It is also used before surgery in patients with locally advanced, inflammatory, or early-stage breast cancer and after surgery in patients with early-stage breast cancer who have a high risk that their cancer will recur (come back). It is also being studied in the treatment of other types of cancer. Perjeta binds to a protein called HER2, which is found on some cancer cells. Blocking this protein may help kill cancer cells.

PET SCAN

A Positron Emission Tomography (PET) scan is an imaging test that helps reveal how your tissues and organs are functioning. A PET scan uses a radioactive drug (tracer) to show this activity.

A PET scan is useful in revealing or evaluating several conditions, including many cancers, heart disease and brain disorders. Often, PET images are combined with CT or MRI scans to create special views.

PROPHYLACTIC MASTECTOMY

Surgery to remove one or both breasts to reduce the risk of developing breast cancer. According to the National Cancer Institute, prophylactic mastectomy in women who carry a BRCA1 or BRCA2 gene mutation may be able to reduce the risk of developing breast cancer by 95%.

STAGE 0

This stage describes cancer in situ, which means "in place." Stage 0 cancers are still located in the place they started and have not spread to nearby tissues. This stage of cancer is often highly curable, usually by removing the entire tumor with surgery.

STAGE I

This stage is usually a small cancer or tumor that has not grown deeply into nearby tissues. It also has not spread to the lymph nodes or other parts of the body. It is often called early-stage cancer.

STAGE II AND III

In general, these 2 stages indicate larger cancers or tumors that have grown more deeply into nearby tissue. They may have also spread to lymph nodes but not to other parts of the body.

STAGE IV

This stage means that the cancer has spread to other organs or parts of the body. It may also be called advanced or metastatic cancer.

TAMOXIFEN (NOLVADEX)

A hormone therapy drug (taken in pill form) used to treat early and advanced stage breast cancers that are hormone receptor-positive. These breast cancers need estrogen to grow. Tamoxifen stops or slows the growth of these tumors by blocking estrogen from attaching to hormone receptors in the cancer cells.

TAXOL

Taxol is an anti-cancer ("antineoplastic" or "cytotoxic") chemotherapy drug. Taxol is classified as a "plant alkaloid," a "taxane" and an "antimicrotubule agent."

TISSUE EXPANDERS

Tissue expanders are temporary, empty implants that are gradually inflated with saline over time. This stretches the skin (and muscle if the expander is placed under the muscle) to make room for the breast implants.

TRIPLE NEGATIVE BREAST CANCER

A breast cancer that is estrogen receptor-negative, progesterone receptor-negative and HER2-negative. This type of breast cancer may grow more quickly than hormone receptor-positive disease, and chemotherapy may work better as a treatment. Inflammatory breast cancer is often triple negative.

VENA CAVA

A large vein that carries blood to the heart from other areas of the body. The vena cava has two parts: the superior vena cava and the inferior vena cava. The superior vena cava carries blood from the head, neck, arms, and chest. The inferior vena cava carries blood from the legs, feet, and organs in the abdomen and pelvis. The vena cava is the largest vein in the body.

Julie Pershing

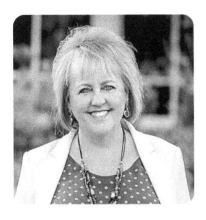

Julie Pershing is an author, book writing coach, and the founder of Gallivant Press.

As a writing coach, Julie helps with all aspects of book writing; from creating your book concept to writing, editing, and successfully publishing your book.

Julie and her husband Dave live in the beautiful Pacific Northwest with their two dogs, Audrey and Everly.

It's not easy to write your story, especially when you are writing about something as personal and life-changing as a cancer diagnosis. I am so grateful the women in this book said yes.

Your story matters. If you are ready to write a book, I would love to be a part of your journey.

Connect with Julie:
Email: hello@gallivantpress.com
Facebook: The Writer Experience
Website: https://gallivantpress.com/
Website: https://juliepershing.com/

Free 30 minute consultation:
https://gallivantpress.as.me/consult

ALSO BY JULIE PERSHING

Waves of Pink: Stories of Sisterhood

Waves of Pink II: Common Ground, Uncommon Courage

Profound Impact: Forging Success Beyond Circumstance

BOOKS FOR ENTREPRENEURS

Focus on Networking

Focus on Speaking

Focus on Coaching

Focus on Systems

Easy eBook: How to Write an ebook in Seven Days

COMING SOON

Focus on Marketing

The Secret We Keep: Breaking the Silence About Domestic Abuse

WRITING AND BOOK COACHING

www.juliepershing.com

DOES YOUR GROUP OR NON-PROFIT WANT TO PUBLISH A BOOK?

Email: hello@gallivantpress.com

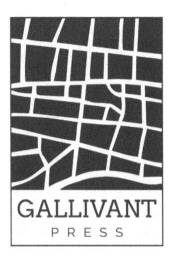

GALLIVANT

P R E S S

It's time to share your story

We're here to help you,
every step of the way

hello@gallivantpress.com
www.gallivantpress.com

CPSIA information can be obtained
at www.ICGtesting.com
Printed in the USA
FSHW022126120421
80416FS